A CUP OF COF|

10 LEADING CHIROPRACTORS IN THE UNITED STATES

VALUABLE INSIGHTS YOU SHOULD
KNOW ABOUT HOW CHIROPRACTIC CARE
CAN IMPROVE YOUR HEALTH

David Friedman, D.C.
Randy Van Ittersum

Rutherford Publishing House
PO Box 969
Ramseur, NC 27316
www.RutherfordPublishingHouse.com

Cover photo: Wavebreak Media Ltd & mjp/Bigstock.com

ISBN-10: 0692372806
ISBN-13: 978-0692372807

TABLE OF CONTENTS

ACKNOWLEDGEMENTS

We all want to thank our husbands and wives, fathers and mothers, and everybody who has played a role in shaping our lives and our attitudes.

To all the clients we've had the honor of working with, who shaped our understanding of the difficulty of this time for you and your families. It has been our privilege to serve each and every one of you.

INTRODUCTION

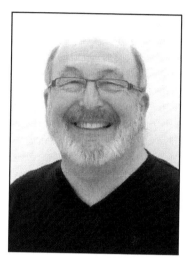

Contributing Author:
Randy Van Ittersum
*Host & Founder – Business
Leader Spotlight Show*

Today's chiropractor may be dubbed the "New Hero" in healthcare in the 21st century. Preventive healthcare didn't start with Patient Protection and Affordable Care Act (PPACA) better known as Obama Care, but this legislation put a new focus on preventive medicine. Its premise is simple; see a doctor before you have acute medical problems. It is a well-known fact that if most medical problems can be identified and treated early, at their onset, one can avoid chronic illness that's then expensive to treat.

Chiropractic care is about "preventive care" and helping your body do what it was designed to do, which is to take care of itself naturally. This is not to say that family physicians and medical specialists are not doing their best to help you, but in the daily course of things, their focus is less on prevention than it is on dealing with chronic illness. Due to the number of patients that family physicians must see in a day and the reimbursement incentives that they are paid by HMO's, a family physician simply doesn't have time to focus on one's overall health. Instead, they must focus on one's current chronic condition.

Although I'm not a doctor, I am surrounded by medical professionals. In my family and extended family, there are seven doctors, a nurse, and a pharmacist. When you consider what they face with government regulations, HMO's and insurance companies, and the sheer number of patients they must treat every day, you quickly understand why they don't have time to focus their attention on diet, exercise, and lifestyle, which are all factors that play a role in one's health.

Although surrounded by well-trained medical people in my family, I also go to a local chiropractor in my community, a doctor by the name of Mark Brusveen D.C. As you read this book, you will begin to understand what I have discovered, which is how chiropractic care can help your health. In fact, in this book we have brought together 10 of America's leading chiropractors to share with you their insights into chiropractic care and the effect it can have on your health.

It is important that you understand that I am now 65 years old, and that I had a major heart attack when I was 42, which was initially treated by having a triple bypass. The damage to my heart left me with only 60% of my heart muscle working, yet I'm still active and ride my bicycle 30-60 minutes, seven days a week. I have a personal physician who is an Internist with a PhD. in medicine, a cardiologist whom I credit with saving my life, three children and their spouses who are doctors, nurses, pharmacist, and my "chiropractor." All of these people play a role in my healthcare.

The goal of this book is to help you understand how chiropractic care can affect your health and why a chiropractor should be one of your primary caregivers. Pain is one of the most common reasons that people go to see a chiropractor. The benefits of chiropractic treatment can be remarkable. You will read stories that clearly show the help that chiropractic care can bring to you.

A lack of pain doesn't necessarily mean that a person is healthy. Most of the time heart disease will not exhibit any symptoms until you experience a heart attack. Eighty percent of the initial phases of cancer are painless until the cancer metastasizes to an organ or bone. The fact is, in the same way that you should maintain the engine in your car, you should maintain your central nervous system. It controls everything. It is crucial to maintain one's spine because it encases and protects the central nervous system.

The philosophy of chiropractic care is that the human body is self-healing and self-repairing. Surgery may be required in some cases, but it's astonishing how many people achieve the same or better outcomes through chiropractic care. In General Spine News in May of 2013, it is reported that for patients who first consulted a surgeon for their condition, 42.7 percent wound up having surgery, compared to 1.5 percent who first consulted a chiropractor. Although you might be skeptical about going to a chiropractor, when you consider the facts as illustrated by the figures above, it would behoove anyone with back problems to see a chiropractor first.

To further support the idea that chiropractic care can have a significant impact on your health, one only needs to turn to a seven-year study posted by the Journal of Physiological and Manipulative Therapeutics involving 70,000 people. The report found that when a person's primary health care provider was a chiropractor, they used 85 percent fewer medications and had 62 percent fewer hospital admissions.

This is not to say that chiropractors know everything about the human body. Our bodies are amazing, and we are learning more about them every day. The human brain controls billions of chemical impulses every second. If you attached every capillary, artery, and vein end to end they would stretch 60,000 miles. The human body is so complex that it is impossible for the medical community to understand it completely.

As a consumer of health care, what is most important is to identify a philosophy of how you want to be treated. We know that your diet, your current lifestyle, your occupation, and psychosocial considerations all have a bearing on your health. Do you want to treat your health with medications and surgeries, or by a drug-free, surgery-free, non-invasive discipline, which is provided through chiropractic care.

Randy Van Ittersum
Host & Founder – Business Leader Spotlight Show

1

CHIROPRACTIC CARE – TREATMENT BEYOND SYMPTOM RELIEF

by David Friedman, D.C.

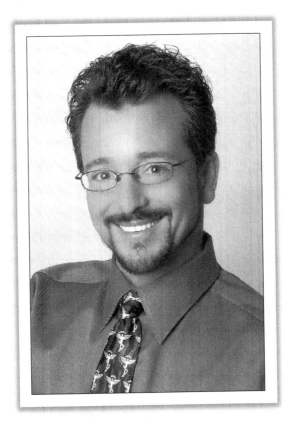

David Friedman, D.C.
Friedman Chiropractic
Wilmington, North Carolina
www.wilmingtonchiropractor.com

Dr. David Friedman is a Chiropractic Physician and certified Doctor of Naturopathy. He received a post-doctorate certification from Harvard Medical School and is a former teacher of Neurology. Dr. Friedman is often referred to as the "Chiropractor to the Stars," as his list of patients includes some of today's top celebrities and movie stars. As "The Health Expert" for Lifetime Television's morning show and host of a syndicated talk radio show, he shares cutting edge health segments with millions of people every week.

Dr. Friedman is a board qualified Chiropractic Neurologist and a member of the American Chiropractic Association, Naturopathic Medical Association, American Dietetic Association and is a registered Naturopathic Diplomate (RND). Friedman Chiropractic has been honored in the National Who's Who Directory for Distinguished Businesses since 2002.

CHIROPRACTIC CARE – TREATMENT BEYOND SYMPTOM RELIEF

For most people, the word "chiropractor" conjures images of having your "back cracked." And while chiropractors do primarily focus on adjusting (realigning) the vertebrae of the back and neck, they also diagnose, treat, and prevent mechanical disorders of the entire musculoskeletal system. From your wrists (carpal tunnel syndrome) and elbows (tendonitis) to the hip (bursitis) and the jaw (TMJ disorders), chiropractors can restore functionality and relieve pain. It's also not uncommon for patients to be treated for back pain and experience improvement in other areas of the body. That's because the spine is the central place through which all nerves travel to your organs, glands, and muscles. For this reason, chiropractors are able to restore proper spinal nerve flow, which allows you to reach your optimal health.

Because chiropractic is a drug-free, surgery-free, non-invasive profession, some people don't consider us to be "real" doctors. Thanks to the multi-billion dollar pharmaceutical industry, prescription drugs have become the go-to "treatment" for inflammation, muscle spasms, aches, and pains. It's quite unfortunate since this leads many people to assume they need the expertise of medical doctors, when, in actuality, chiropractors are required to have the same medical courses and study from the exact text books that primary physicians use during their training. When you look at total classroom hours, chiropractors lead the way and are even required to perform more cadaver dissections than medical doctors. While MDs have advanced training in chemistry, surgery, and pharmacology, chiropractors receive more education in anatomy, physiology, neurology, and x-ray. It takes eight years of college education to become a doctor of chiropractic and, just as MDs can become specialists in their field, chiropractors can also earn advanced degrees in orthopedics, neurology, sports medicine, and pediatrics. After graduating, I went through an additional three years of college training to earn my post-doctorate degree in neurology. Chiropractic was once the best-kept secret in health care; however, that's rapidly changing. Chiropractic is now part of the mainstream medical system and covered by all major health insurances, Medicare, Medicaid, and workers' compensation. Many chiropractors practice in the same office with medical doctors and in some states, chiropractors have hospital privileges. Chiropractic is the safest drug-free, non-invasive therapy for the treatment of back, neck, and other musculoskeletal problems.

Some people who have never been to a chiropractor have a fear of the unknown and are concerned about the safety of spinal adjustments. I can attest that when performed by licensed chiropractors, spinal adjustments are *extremely* safe. Consider this: in one lifetime, people have a better chance of being struck three times by lightning than ever being injured by a chiropractor. Many people feel safe taking over-the-counter pain medications, yet these come with serious side effects. Recent research shows that the two most popular over-the-counter painkillers have potentially fatal risks. Taking ibuprofen for a long period of time can lead to kidney dysfunction, stroke, and heart attack[1]. Daily use of acetaminophen, could lead to permanent liver damage. Tens of thousands of Americans are hospitalized each year for liver problems caused by acetaminophen and many die[2]. While medications can often do wonders at *masking* symptoms, chiropractors safely *treat* the cause of your ailments.

MOMS, BABIES, AND CHILDREN

If you are pregnant, plan to be pregnant, or know somebody with such aspirations, chiropractic care is the safest drug-free method of choice for health care during pregnancy. According to research published in the *Journal of Chiropractic Medicine*[3], pregnant mothers who engage in regular chiropractic care show reduced back pain during pregnancy and less labor time, making delivery easier and less traumatic for themselves and for their babies. Maintaining proper pelvic alignment during the gestation period helps to increase the amount of room available for the baby in the womb and helps preserve the normal nerve flow from the lumbar spine to the uterus. The increased weight during pregnancy can often lead to lower back pain and sciatica (leg pain). Since it's advised not to take medicine during pregnancy, chiropractic is the natural solution. In my office, I use a special chiropractic table that opens up to accommodate a larger belly, so we can adjust an expectant mom during all phases of her pregnancy.

If the delivery is overdue and the doctor is considering inducing labor, a simple chiropractic adjustment will often do the trick without the need for labor-inducing drugs. Several OB/GYN doctors in my town refer their patients to my office before resorting to inducing labor.

For whatever reason, some babies seem determined to enter the world in the breech position—backward, with their buttocks and legs appearing where the head should be. Before opting for a C-section, the recommended procedure for breech babies, expectant mothers should find a chiropractor who performs the Webster Technique: an adjustment that actually turns the infant within the womb. This procedure has been clinically shown to achieve an 82 percent success rate of turning babies to their normal position after the eighth month of pregnancy[4]! The Webster Technique not only helps to balance a pregnant woman's pelvis, it also reduces undue stress to her uterus and supporting ligaments. More importantly, it isn't invasive or risk-prone like a C-section, or any other surgical procedure.

I treated a patient named Susan, who was pregnant with her fifth child. I adjusted her regularly during this pregnancy. She did not have chiropractic care during her previous pregnancies, which all had an average labor time of twenty hours. One day she called my office to say her water had broken, and she was on her way. "Congratulations! Call us when you give birth," my office manager said.

Susan replied, "When I said I'm on my way, I mean I'm on my way to *your office*, so I can get one more adjustment before I give birth."

My office manager came running to me in a panic. "Should I boil some water?"

Susan arrived and I gave her one more treatment before she went to the hospital. Susan gave birth to a baby boy within an hour after her leaving my office.

Susan's OB/GYN, who had delivered all of her other children, asked her how she had such a smooth birth compared to all the others, and Susan informed him that she had been receiving regular chiropractic care. Since then, her doctor has referred dozens of pregnant patients to me. Just to be clear, my office manager hasn't yet been required to boil water or assist in any deliveries. Chiropractors are required to have classroom training in childbirth, this is not a procedure we are licensed to perform, nor do we want to. However, we can certainly help the birth process go much more smoothly.

When looking at some of the complications to a child during birth, forceps delivery is at the top of the list. When forceps are used, up to 40 pounds of pressure is applied to the baby's head and neck while being pulled out. It's difficult to imagine that kind of force on an infant, who only weighs between six and eight pounds. When you inflict pressure that is equivalent to three to four times his body weight on a tiny little head and neck, there can be serious consequences.

Furthermore, pulling with so much pressure on an infant's head can cause injury to the vertebra and phrenic nerve, which supplies nerve flow to the heart and lungs. When the phrenic nerve in the neck is irritated, it compromises the diaphragm and makes breathing more difficult. Research published in the *Journal of Forensic Science* shows that this can even lead to sudden infant death syndrome.[5] So, when a chiropractor adjusts the mother's pelvic during gestation, this makes room for the infant and significantly reduces the need for forceps during delivery. Including chiropractic care before, during, and after pregnancy is a win-win for infant and mom.

AS THE TWIG IS BENT, SO GROWS THE TREE

I'm a firm believer in getting children checked by a chiropractor. Just as parents take their child to the family MD for wellness visits and to the dentist for regular oral checkups, bringing a child to a chiropractor is also a good idea. If any issues are found, just a few treatments can often help your child's "crooked twig" grow into a healthy tree. Adjusting a child's spine is like working on soft, moist clay instead of trying to remold clay that is already hardened, as is the case with adults. I enjoy seeing children because results occur so quickly. Children with certain conditions (e.g., asthma, colic, bed-wetting, and scoliosis) respond wonderfully to chiropractic care.[6] However, I see the greatest results in children when it comes to ear infections (otitis media). Almost half of all children will get a middle ear infection before they're a year old, and sixty-six percent will have an ear infection by the age of three.[7] Frequent ear infections are the second most common reason for surgery in children. Circumcision, by the way, is the first.

Typically, medical doctors want to go the antibiotic route when treating ear infections. Thankfully, the practice of regularly prescribing children antibiotics is currently under fire. Just break down the word and you can see why. The definition of the word *anti* means "against"; the word *biotic* means "life." So the actual definition of antibiotic is "against life" (i.e., death!). While these drugs indeed kill off bad bacteria in the body, prolonged use can destroy a child's good flora of bacteria, which is needed for optimal health. Frequent antibiotic use in children has been linked to increased risk of childhood obesity and type 2 diabetes[8] , and the development of resistant bacteria—microorganisms that don't respond to antibiotics that may have worked in the past.[9]

If antibiotics don't work for your child's ear infection, the doctor will drill tiny holes in his or her eardrum and insert tubes to drain the fluid from the ear canal (eustachian tube) and call this "mission accomplished." However, these treatments don't address the cause of the problem. Puncturing a child's eardrum also leaves scar tissue, which can lead to partial deafness. When a chiropractor sees children for ear infections, he will adjust the cervical spine, which can improve the function of the cervical ganglion located between the first and fourth bone in the neck. Doing this allows the eustachian tube in the ear to better drain excess fluid from the middle ear, build up its own antibodies, and recover more quickly[10]. In addition to chiropractic care, it's important for children suffering from ear infections to stop ingesting dairy products because this creates mucus build up inside the sinuses and ears, which can contribute to ear infections.

The second ailment that responds well to chiropractic care is colic.[11] One of my female patients, who was being treated for headaches, came in one day and looked just awful! She had dark circles under her bloodshot eyes. She had a six-week-old newborn who kept her up night after night due to colic.

"Why don't you bring in your baby and let me check his spine?" I asked her.
"Well, isn't he too little and fragile to be adjusted?" she asked.

"No," I said. "I don't adjust a child like I adjust you. It's very gentle. We can correct misalignments, which can relieve the colic."

The day after she brought in the baby for his adjustment, she called to tell me that she'd enjoyed her first full night of sleep in six weeks. She was so excited, she actually urged other mothers in her music-play group who had colicky babies to come see me. For parents who have a colicky baby and want a good night's sleep, visiting a chiropractor is a great, and little known, solution!

ADJUSTING HEROES ON THE HALF SHELL...

I have had the opportunity to treat people from all walks of life, including some of today's top A-list celebrities. In 1989, I began working on the movie *Teenage Mutant Ninja Turtles* after one of the leading turtles hurt his back during a martial arts scene. As the years progressed, I went from a Turtle to Travolta. It's not uncommon for cast and crew to work long, sixteen- to eighteen-hour days. The film industry has learned to rely on chiropractic care to get their actors and crew through those long days and nights of standing, bending, and lifting. When chiropractors are involved in a film, they usually see most of the cast and crew—from the camera men and makeup artists to the directors and actors. When a film sets up on location, one of the first things on a production coordinator's list is to find a good chiropractor for the cast and crew. Over the years, I've been blessed to be on that list.

...AND OTHER NATIONAL TREASURES

I live in Wilmington, North Carolina, home of Screen Gems Studio. When movies and TV productions are being filmed in our city, such as the *Matlock* series starring Andy Griffith, I am often asked to take care of the cast and crew. By the end of the first season of *Matlock*, I was providing chiropractic care to the whole gang with one exception—the star of the show. Andy adamantly refused to see a chiropractor! His co-workers said that he had a bad experience with a chiropractor decades earlier and had sworn never to see another one. In fact, he would even make fun of the rest of the cast and crew for coming to see me.

One evening during the second season, while watching an episode of *Matlock*, I noticed a scene in which Andy appeared to be in pain. The next day I mentioned this to Frank Thackery, one of the directors of the series. Two hours later my office phone rang—Andy Griffith was calling to make an appointment. He said that if his pain was so apparent that acting couldn't even cover it up, then he needed to get relief right away!

Unlike many of the celebrities who arrive at my office by chauffeur-driven limo or sneak in and out of the back door, Andy drove himself to the office in a Ford pickup. He walked into the waiting room and announced to my receptionist, "My name's Andy Griffith, and I'm here to see Dr. Friedman." He then proceeded to spell his last name, humbly assuming she wouldn't know who he was. Since *The Andy Griffith Show* was based on the life of a man in a tiny North Carolina town called Mayberry, there's not a person in my state who doesn't know this iconic man.

After examination and x-rays, I gave Andy an adjustment. He walked out of my office so happy and with such relief from his symptoms, the next day he referred his wife, Cindy, to see me. His co-workers told me that Andy's demeanor changed after receiving chiropractic adjustments. He would literally sing and whistle (just like on his show) on the days following his treatments.

As we were approaching the 100th anniversary of Chiropractic, I thought about how wonderful it would be to have Andy Griffith on the cover of *Today's Chiropractic Magazine*, commemorating this special time in the history of our field. Along with baseball and apple pie, the name Andy Griffith has always been considered an all-American treasure. So, I asked Cindy if she thought her husband would be interested in allowing me to interview him? She told me that since gossip and controversy seems to be what sells in the media, he didn't want to be misquoted or misrepresented, so Andy rarely granted interviews. Nevertheless, I worked up the courage to ask him if he would grant me the honor of an interview. He accepted, and I was humbled by his reason. He told me he wanted to give back to the profession that made such a positive impact on his life.

After the article had been published, I received thousands of thank you letters from chiropractors across the country. The article increased awareness of chiropractic care among senior citizens tenfold and gave it the credibility it deserved! At that time, *Matlock* was the number one show on television in that market, and there could not have been a better endorsement for chiropractic care than a member of that very generation, Andy Griffith. In fact, I had pleaded with my grandmother for many years to see a chiropractor, to no avail. After sending her the article, she called me to say that she was seeing a chiropractor and was already feeling so much better.

"I'm your grandson, and I've been asking you for years to go see a chiropractor!" I could hear the smile in her voice as she replied, "Yes. You are my grandson, and I love you to death, but *he's Andy Griffith.*"

I would later have Andy as a guest on my syndicated radio show, when he granted me another rare opportunity for a candid interview. I wasn't nervous until right before we went live on the air. Andy said to me, "David, the last time I granted an interview was over ten years ago to Larry King." I didn't fill Larry's shoes that day, but the interview still came off very well. May you rest in peace, dear friend.

HEALING THE WHOLE HOUSE

When you purchase a house and hire a home inspector to assess its condition, he or she will examine the home's foundation, crawlspace, floors, walls, ceilings, and attic. This provides a total picture of the health of the house. I believe that the same considerations hold true when a patient comes to see me. From the foundation (your feet) to the head (your ceiling), everything is connected. If there's a problem with the foundation, it can affect the alignment of the walls, which can throw your ceiling off-center. While it's important to maintain a normal alignment of the spine, I believe for proper functionality, it's just as important to assess the extremities.

I treated a woman who had chronic low back pain, who one day mentioned that she had reoccurring heel spurs on her right foot. Within a year of having them surgically removed, the spur would grow back. When I examined her, I noticed she leaned to the right when she was standing. After talking with her, I discovered that her heel spur always developed on the right side and that she had injured her left knee playing volleyball years before. After that injury, she avoided pain by favoring the other side when she walked, which put too much weight on the right foot. Voila! The cause of her heel spur was uncovered. I adjusted her left knee twice a week for about three weeks, and soon, she was able to walk without favoring one side. No more knee pain and no more spurs, just because I examined and treated something she hadn't considered—her knee.

I'll share another example of the importance of treating extremities. A professional golfer came in to see me suffering from epicondylitis, sometimes referred to as "golfer's elbow." The pain was so intense that he had undergone several cortisone shots, physical therapy, and anti-inflammatory drugs. He also tried massage therapy and chiropractic care for his neck. While these attempts did relieve some of his symptoms, he was still not able to play golf without elbow pain. When I met him, he was thinking about throwing in the towel and giving up on golf, which as a professional golfer and instructor, would have been financially devastating for him. After I had examined him, it was obvious that the bone in his elbow (called the radial head) wasn't moving properly, which was causing inflammation and pain every time he swung a golf club. Using my hand, I made a quick, painless thrust and realigned his elbow, and he experienced immediate relief. He is now pain-free and back on the golf course.

CARPAL TUNNEL SYNDROME

On the subject of extremities, carpal tunnel syndrome is hands-down (pun intended) one of my favorite ailments to treat. Symptoms include pain, tingling, and numbness in the wrist and the hand. Neck alignments can help the nerve signals flow better to the hands, but complete relief of carpal tunnel requires examination and gentle realignment of the bones in the wrist.

During my exam, I do pre and post grip strength tests, and the results after treatment are phenomenal! I have seen patients, who had no strength at all in their hands that are able to open a pickle jar after their adjustment. Sometimes, I'll recommend a wrist brace and exercises for my patients, and review ways that the hands can be used without aggravating the condition. Apart from typing and hammering, there can be other activities that compound these problems. For example, pushing things with the wrist in an extended position, like giving somebody a high five, aggravates carpal tunnel. I tell patients suffering from carpal tunnel, "use your fist to close doors." When pushing yourself up from a chair, use your fist instead of the extended hand. That one tip alone will help you more than you can imagine. From a nutritional point of view, eat pineapples, because they contain an enzyme called bromelain, which helps to reduce inflammation of the wrist. In summertime, enjoy watermelons. They act as a diuretic, which can reduce swelling in the wrist and give great results for those suffering with carpal tunnel syndrome.

TMJ DYSFUNCTION

The temporomandibular joint (TMJ) is essentially a hinge that connects the jaw to the temporal bones of your skull. This joint allows the jaw to move up and down and side to side, so you can talk, chew, and yawn. Disorders of the TMJ can be caused or affected by teeth-grinding, jaw-clenching, dental work, trauma, and even stress. The most common symptoms are clicking, popping, or grating sounds that happen when you open or close your mouth to chew. This may or may not be painful. Sometimes, a dysfunction of the jaw just makes popping sounds, but I've also seen TMJ cause debilitating headaches, hearing loss, dizziness, and ringing in the ears.

There's an easy test you can do to determine whether or not you have TMJ dysfunction. Place each of your index fingers on the side of your face, immediately in front of your ear. When you open and close your mouth, these joints should move together. If one moves before the other, you have a TMJ issue. In my office, I use a very gentle, pain-free technique that realigns the joint. Relief is usually achieved within minutes. It's that dramatic.

One of my favorite TMJ success stories involved a patient, who came into the office one day because she was experiencing headaches. When I weighed this 5-foot-2-inch woman, I was appalled to learn that she weighed eighty-eight pounds! She said that she had lost thirty-five pounds over the past year due to pain in her mouth, which prevented her from eating. She opened her mouth, removed her dentures, and showed me several raw ulcers on her gums. She had visited three dentists, and even went to a dental teaching institute, thinking she'd have better luck there after having her dentures refit and then readjusted. Nothing helped.

While she was telling this story, I could hear an odd popping sound. "Was that your jaw that just popped?" I asked her.

"Oh yeah," she told me. "It's been doing that since a car accident I had two years ago."

When I checked her jaw alignment, I discovered that she had severe TMJ dysfunction. This was affecting her bite, which is why her dentures didn't fit properly. I realigned her jaw. She immediately closed her mouth, and tears started rolling down her cheeks. She told me that it was the first time in over a year that her dentures had lined up without causing pain. All of the prior specialists she had visited were so busy checking the alignment of her dentures that they failed to look beyond the symptoms and examine the joint that controls chewing. Within three months of that simple adjustment, she was back to a healthy 120 pounds, because she was finally able to eat without pain. Oh, and the headaches she had come to see me for were also related to her TMJ dysfunction and completely resolved under care.

SHOULDER PROBLEMS

Robert has been a patient of mine for more than ten years and has experienced great success under my care for chronic lower back pain. Because he does construction work for a living, he comes in every four to six weeks for a spinal "tune-up." During one of his appointments, Robert told me he was stressing about having to miss two months of work after next week's shoulder surgery for his torn rotator cuff. I asked him why he never mentioned to me that he had a shoulder problem? He replied, "I thought you only worked on people's backs?"

I examined his shoulder and felt it was something I could treat. Robert canceled his surgery, and I put him on a treatment plan which included shoulder adjustments and exercises. In less than a month, Robert's shoulder was as good as new without any drugs or surgery, and he didn't miss a single day of work.

While chiropractors can't mend a "torn" ligament or tendon, we can restore proper alignment of the joint surrounding the tear, which increases motion, blood, and nerve flow to an area, making it more conducive to healing. Think of a door that has three hinge joints. If one of these hinges came loose, the door would no longer open and close properly. This "misaligned" door would squeak when you opened and closed it and rub against the wooden door frame, causing wear and tear.

Likewise, when a shoulder joint is not aligned properly, this can cause wear and tear on the ligaments and tendons. Since Robert's experience, I now make it a point to ask all my patients regularly to let me know if there's anything bothering them *beside their back and neck.*

DIET AND NUTRITION

I've seen a remarkable difference in the success rates between patients who eat healthy foods and take natural supplements, compared to those who don't. "You are what you eat" definitely applies to your spine, discs, muscles, and ligaments. For example, if you're suffering from muscle spasms and drinking a lot of milk, I can treat you for weeks, but I won't be able to help you. Dairy products offer a lousy source of calcium and contain a protein called casein, which can lead to inflammation of the joints and muscle spasms, or "Charlie horses" in your legs and feet.

Additionally, it's not uncommon to see patients arrive with a stuffy nose, get a neck adjustment, and leave my office breathing perfectly. However, if a patient is eating a lot of peanut butter, this could create mucus build-up, leaving him more prone to sinus infections. One of my patients suffered from chronic sinus problems for many years. She tried every nose spray, pill, herbal tea, and sought care from two chiropractors. I did something a little different; I asked about her diet. She told me, her favorite thing to eat at night was a peanut butter sandwich. After suggesting that she might have a dormant peanut allergy, I recommended that she switch to almond butter, and she did. Two weeks later, the sinus problems were gone. If I had solely adjusted her spine, I would have been just as unsuccessful in alleviating her sinus problem as everything and everyone else.

I'm also an advocate of whole food nutritional supplements, because you don't have to worry about overdosing or having negative reactions. Since the human body wasn't created in a laboratory, adding synthetic elements to nutritional products can contribute to disease and create other antagonistic effects. For example, researchers at Johns Hopkins report that taking vitamin E supplements, in excess of 400 IU, is associated with a higher overall risk of death![12] However, natural sources of vitamin E (wheat germ, nuts, seeds, olives, spinach, asparagus, and green leafy vegetables) are not harmful and are needed by the body.

The most popular nutritional supplement on the market is vitamin C (ascorbic acid). What people don't realize is very few vitamin C supplements on the store shelves come from natural sources. They are made from the same chemicals used to make nail polish remover (acetone); gasoline (benzene), paint (toluene), and toilet bowl cleaner (bleach!) Research from Mount Sinai School of Medicine has shown that vitamin C supplements cause genetic damage to humans. Does that mean vitamin C is bad for you? No, the nutrient is vital to our survival; we just need to look to nature for it, not chemists. You get more than enough vitamin C from foods like citrus fruits, red sweet peppers, kiwi, strawberries, and Brussels sprouts.

Having a degree in naturopathy, which utilizes a holistic nutritional approach to healing and disease prevention, I spent several years formulating all-natural whole food chewable products, which are sold around the world. These products don't contain harmful chemicals, binders, coloring agents, artificial sweeteners, or preservatives. They offer optimal nutritional support to all generations, from pregnant females and infants to great-grandparents.

SURGERY—THE VERY LAST RESORT

Chiropractors don't put much stock in surgery, until—and unless—it is the only option left. We often see patients who have already tried surgery and were not happy with the results. Sadly, 74 percent of those who undergo spinal surgery will not experience relief of their symptoms.[13] Statistically, those who have a surgically fused vertebra in their spine will undergo two more operations in their lifetime. It's an endless cycle. Fusing vertebrae in the spine makes the vertebra above work harder causing it to become too mobile (loose.) Eventually, that vertebra malfunctions, and surgeons want to fuse it to the vertebra above that one, which makes the segment above that one too mobile, and so on. This common occurrence is known as "failed back surgery syndrome".

It baffles me how many people believe back surgery is effective and safe, but they're afraid to go to a chiropractor. Unlike surgeons, chiropractors will not make you sign a waiver before a procedure that asks you to acknowledge all of the dangerous risks involved. That's because having chiropractic care, unlike surgery, does not pose the risk of nerve damage, paralysis, brain damage, or death.

Chiropractic care is the most conservative spinal treatment option in the world. It should be the first on your list before ever considering going under the knife.

ANSWERS TO COMMONLY ASKED QUESTIONS

Over the past twenty-five years, I've been asked an array of questions about chiropractic care. The following are answers to some of the more common ones.

What is an adjustment?

An adjustment is another name for a realignment of a joint. Simply put, we apply a very specific force to a joint that's not moving properly. This safe and natural procedure will improve spinal function, eliminate nerve interference, and support overall health.

Do adjustments hurt?

Most chiropractic techniques use minimal force. Patients can very often experience pain relief after just one treatment. Any initial soreness or increased pain following an adjustment would be similar to feeling sore after starting an exercise program.

What is that popping sound that I sometimes hear during an adjustment?

Those popping sounds are tiny pockets of air being released in the joint. A chiropractic adjustment takes the pressure off of the connective tissue that holds the joint together. Basically, you are hearing an air bubble being released, like the popping sound that happens when you poke the little air bubbles in plastic packing sheets.

My mother told me that cracking my knuckles will give me arthritis. Is that true?

Actually, that's an old wives' tale—probably created by annoyed parents. Research has indicated that knuckle cracking actually prevents arthritis because it creates more movement inside the joint.[14] Arthritis, on the other hand, causes a lack of movement inside of a joint.

Is it better to wait until you're in pain to visit a chiropractor?
Pain brings most people into my office, yet pain is almost always the last symptom to show up. Just like you can have a cavity inside a tooth for years and not know it, only to bite into a piece of candy and experience pain, the same holds true for your body. Some of my patients have felt fine, bent over to tie their shoes, and suddenly suffered debilitating back pain. It wasn't an act of tying their shoes, but the lack of prevention on their part that led to the symptom of pain. Just like people shouldn't wait until smoke comes out of their car engine before bringing it to a mechanic, having chiropractic checkups, before experiencing pain, will keep your spine in check.

Once you start treatments, do you have to keep seeing a chiropractor forever?
In my office, pain relief can usually be achieved within a couple weeks of care (or nine visits). If a structural component needs to be addressed, corrective care can take an additional eight weeks. This time frame is similar to the healing span of a sprained ankle or joint, which usually takes eight weeks to mend. Afterward, patients go on a maintenance regimen, which is similar to going to your dentist for regular teeth cleanings and checkups. This phase varies. A sedentary eighty-year-old may need to see me once every month because of his inactivity. An active young man who is exposed to more physical stress like lifting heavy sheetrock might also need to see me once a month. I have some patients who need maintenance treatments twice a year. Genetics, lack of exercise, and common daily activities (sitting, posture, sleeping habits) also play a role

when determining the length of time that one's body can last between chiropractic treatments.

Since a spinal adjustment takes twenty minutes or less, this leaves you with twenty-three hours and forty minutes in your day. If you spend eight of those hours slouching over a desk at work or sleeping wrong, this can undo the effect of the wonderful chiropractic treatments you received. I believe regular maintenance is critical for overall wellness and to keep the pain from returning. Seeing a chiropractor to maintain the corrective care you receive is similar to wearing a retainer or seeing your orthodontist for occasional checkups after your teeth are straightened. The good news is while it takes an orthodontist two to three years to straighten teeth, chiropractic care can take just two to three months to straighten the spine. The worst scenario I see is when a happy patient comes back after a year or two, with the exact same symptoms, because he failed to get spinal tune-ups every few months. Maintenance care is important.

I've tried chiropractic before and didn't get any relief. Why?
The word "chiropractic" literally means "done by hand," and no two hands are exactly alike. If you went to a hairdresser who gave you a lousy haircut, you wouldn't give up on all hairdressers; you'd find another one that gave you the haircut that you wanted. Also, there are different chiropractic tools and techniques. For example, I use a flexion distraction table that does wonders for herniated discs. Some chiropractors don't offer this option to their patients. I also treat carpal tunnel syndrome while some practitioners aren't proficient in treating this condition. So, if you do not see the results that you expect, talk to your chiropractor about trying a different approach or seek care somewhere else.

What is the most common ailment that chiropractors treat?
In the 1990s, the most common condition chiropractors treated was lower back pain. Then came the rise in computer and video game use, so I saw a lot of carpal tunnel syndrome and tendinitis. In the last eight years, the most common condition that I treat is called "text neck." Four billion people own cell phones and constantly use them to send text messages or surf the net. Spending too much time on a smart phone or a computer tablet with your head lowered is now the leading cause of headaches, neck pain, and arm numbness—even in children!

How does texting cause spinal troubles?
Your head weighs about ten pounds. For every inch forward that you slouch, you can add another ten pounds. If you are slouching five inches away from the back of the chair, you have added an additional 50 pounds of pressure to your neck and mid-back area. If you don't stop slouching while texting, this can lead to headaches, neck pain, arm numbness, and even permanent arthritis. On my website www.DoctorDavidFriedman.com, I review a few stretches that can prevent text neck.

How can I find a good chiropractor?
Ask for a referral from a friend, family member, or a fellow coworker. Turn to the people you know and trust. There's no better form of advertising than a satisfied patient.

What makes your work worthwhile?
There is simply no greater reward than the success stories that I hear every week from my patients. From the grandfather with a bad shoulder who is now able to play catch with his grandson, to the athlete with tennis elbow who gets back on the court, to the

older couple who can dance together again, these unforgettable stories make my job a true joy. However, in order to truly appreciate the impact of chiropractic care, I want to share a letter I received from Richard.

Richard came into my office in such agonizing pain that it literally took him thirty minutes to make it from his car to my waiting room. Three years earlier, he was diagnosed with a herniated lumbar disc and had recently undergone back surgery that only offered temporary relief. Prior to his back surgery, he tried medications and pain management. He also saw an orthopedist, a neurologist, and a physical therapist. All of the relief that he attained was short-lived, and afterward, he would end up in excruciating pain. And now he was facing the decision of going for a second surgery! I could relate to Richard's suffering because I too had been diagnosed with a herniated lumbar disc when I was younger. The pain is unrelenting! Thanks to chiropractic care, I was cured, and that experience is the primary reason I became a chiropractor. When I assured Richard that he was in the right place, he rolled his eyes at me. Obviously, he'd heard that one before.

After treating Richard daily in my office for three weeks, he was pain-free and enjoying life again. Richard was just another one of many patients that I'd treated who no longer had back pain, but it wasn't that simple. One day, I received a thank you card from Richard that read:

> *"Dr. Friedman, words cannot describe my gratitude. I didn't tell you something during my consultation. The excruciating pain had gotten so unbearable, I had just purchased a handgun to end it all and put myself out of that misery. I just couldn't live another day in such*

agony! Then a coworker recommended I come see you. Dr. Friedman, you were my last hope; my final attempt to get relief. Your chiropractic treatments brought my back to life and gave me my life back! I thank you. My wife, daughter, and grandchild thank you."

I've never been quite so moved as I was the day that I received that letter from Richard. Pain can affect people's social, family, and work life. For some, it can also strip them of their willpower to wake up and face another day. Pain quite often takes away things most of us take for granted, like our ability to walk. I had an elderly patient named Sally, who required the assistance of a cane in order to walk. With every step, she would groan with pain. I adjusted her for a couple of weeks. One day after she left the office, I returned to the treatment room and noticed Sally's cane leaning against the wall. She had walked out of my office without it! As I looked at her forgotten cane, I couldn't stop grinning. I'm so blessed to be part of a profession that helps add life to people's years and more years to their life.

(This content should be used for informational purposes only. It does not create a doctor-patient relationship with any reader and should not be construed as medical advice. If you need medical advice, please contact a doctor in your community who can assess the specifics of your situation.)

References:

[1]"Ibuprofen Can Triple Stroke Risk; Painkillers Can Double Heart Attack Chances." *Medical News Today*: MediLexicon, Intl., 12 Jan. 2011. Web, 28 Dec. 2014. http://www.medicalnewstoday.com/articles/213506.php.

[2]"Overdoing acetaminophen." *Harvard Medical School Health Guide*: Jun 29, 2009. www.health.harvard.edu/fhg/updates/overdoing-acetaminophen. shtml.

[3]*J Chiropr Med.*: 2007 Spring; 6(2), 70–74. www.ncbi.nlm.nih.gov/pmc/artic les/PMC2647084/.

[4]"The Webster Technique: A chiropractic technique with obstetric implications." *J Manipulative and Physiological Therapy*: Volume 25, Issue 6, July–August 2002. http://www.ncbi.nlm.nih.gov/pubmed/12183701.

[5]"Phrenic nerves and diaphragms in sudden infant death syndrome." *Forensic Science International*: Volume 91, Issue 2, 30 January 1998, Pages 133–146. www.sciencedirect.com/science/article/pii/S0379073897001874.

[6]*Chiropractic Pediatric Research.* www.chiropracticpediatricresearch.net/.

[7]*American Chiropractic Association.* http://www.acatoday.org/content_css.cf m?CID=69.

[8]*JAMA Pediatr.* 2014; 168(11):1063–1069. doi:10.1001/jamapediatrics.2014. 1539. http://archpedi.jamanetwork.com/article.aspx?articleid=1909801.

[9]"The Danger of Antibiotic Overuse" *KidsHealth* http://kidshealth.org/parent/ h1n1_center/h1n1_center_treatment/antibiotic_overuse.html.

[10]"Study and Investigation of Ottis Media in Young Children". *J Chiro Research*: Hendricks, Larkin-Their, Vol 2 Jan 1989

[11]"The Short-Term Effect of Spinal Manipulation in the Treatment of Infantile Colic: A Randomized Controlled Clinical Trial with a Blinded Observer." *Journal of Manipulative and Physiological Therapeutics.* 1999; 22(8): 517–522. http://www.chiro.org/pediatrics/ABSTRACTS/Short_Term_ Effect.shtml.

[12]"High-Dose Vitamin E Supplements May Increase Risk of Dying" *Johns Hopkins Medicine.* November 10, 2004. http://www.hopkinsmedicine.org/pre ss_releases/2004/11_10_04.html.

[13]*Spine*: 15 February 2011, Volume 36, Issue 4, pp 320–331. http://www.chir o.org/LINKS/ABSTRACTS/Long-term_Outcomes_of_Lumbar_Fusion.shtml

[14]"Is Cracking Your Knuckles Bad?" *Time Magazine* Oct. 22, 2014. http://tim e.com/3529225/cracking-knuckles-arthritis/.

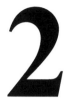

2

INNATE INTELLIGENCE –CHIROPRACTIC AND YOUR ONBOARD HEALING MECHANISMS

by David VanDehey, D.C.

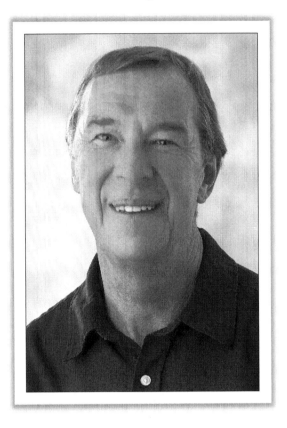

David VanDehey, D.C.
VanDehey Chiropractic
Bourbonnais, Illinois
www.vandeheychiro.com

Dr. David VanDehey is a Chiropractor having attended the Palmer College of Chiropractic. He was inspired by his father, who was an exceptionally gifted chiropractor, to follow in his footsteps.

His philosophy is we all have the God-given right to be healthy; this is possible only through healthy choices.

His upbringing was unique, in that he never received a vaccination, and has never taken medications of any kind in his life. His belief is that health comes from inside the body, never from any medications. His family achieves health through a healthy lifestyle that includes regular chiropractic adjustments, natural whole foods and supplements, staying physically fit by challenging their physical abilities.

INNATE INTELLIGENCE – CHIROPRACTIC AND YOUR ONBOARD HEALING MECHANISMS

The first adjustment formed the chiropractic philosophy. In Davenport, Iowa on September 18, 1895, Dr. Daniel David Palmer (D.D. Palmer) gave the first adjustment to a janitor working in the building in which he practiced. In 1878, the janitor had been stooped over lifting a box when he heard cracking and popping sounds in his neck; he lost his hearing a week later. 17 years after this incident, Dr. Palmer examined the man and found a prominent bony displacement in his neck that was very tender to the touch. Dr. Palmer convinced the man to lay on an exam table. After the adjustment, the man said that his hearing had been restored.

Dr. Palmer stated health is about function and adaptation. This is accomplished through the central nervous system. From that point on, he began to devise a chiropractic philosophy and applied it to people to help them get well naturally—without the use of drugs or surgery. In other words, a natural form of healthcare. That is how our profession began.

The story about how I entered the chiropractic field is very personal. In 1953, my father was attending Palmer College of Chiropractic. That year, my brother Michael was born with a severe case of hydrocephaly. In a normal brain, ventricles produce cerebrospinal fluid that flows from your brain to your spinal cord to nourish and lubricate the spine and the top of the spinal column. In cases of hydrocephaly, the flow is obstructed so that fluid builds up in the brain. At the time of Michael's birth, there were no medical procedures to help with hydro-cephaly. He was just struggling for his life in a hospital room.

Dr. B.J. Palmer, D.D. Palmer's son and a world-renowned leader in the field, heard that one of the students at his college had an infant who had been born with hydrocephaly. Dr. Palmer took my dad out of a class and drove him to the hospital. My dad picked up my brother and carried him out of the hospital. When a doctor told my father that it would be his fault if something happened to Michael, my father said, "Nothing is being done here. We've got to do something."

If my brother had been born today, doctors would insert shunts into the ventricles of the brain to drain the fluid into the stomach. Dr. Palmer took Michael to his clinic (the world-renowned Mayo Clinic of chiropractic care), performed an analysis, and gave him chiropractic adjustments in the upper cervical spine. He gave him adjustments every day for months until eventually the fluid drained out completely. Dr. Palmer saved my brother's life.

When people in the public say that chiropractic care does not work, I tell them that story. The development of chiro-practic care saved my brother's life. Even though he wasn't able to walk until he was three years old, he is now 61 years old and in good health.

THE PHILOSOPHY OF CHIROPRACTIC CARE

The philosophy of chiropractic care is very simple, yet very powerful. Its basic premise is that the human body is self-healing, self-regulating, and self-repairing. All living things have an inborn intelligence from the moment of conception; it exists within our neurological systems and is referred to as "innate intelligence." The function of innate intelligence is to adapt universal forces so that the body coordinates its actions to maintain its existence.

This is the key premise behind chiropractic care. There are 33 basic principles that are centered on natural biological laws and principles. The first major premise is this - there is a universal intelligence in all living matter and continually gives to it all its' properties and actions, thus maintaining it in existence. The other 32 principles revolve around this philosophy. Dr. Palmer taught, almost 100 years ago, that there is a tone or a vibration within the neurological system. If the tone is the correct frequency, you will have good health. It took many years of research to find that stress breaks down the human body and directly impacts the functions of our neurological system. The three sources of stress are emotional, chemical, and physical. These stresses cause disturbances and interferences within the neurological system, so that your body doesn't function well, cannot adapt well, and begins to break down and produce symptoms.

Encountering a stressor that is greater than our body's ability to adapt, whether it is chemical, physical, or emotional, it can lead to a short-circuit in the body's neurological system. When the system becomes over-stimulated, the muscles begin to tense and tighten up; they are out of balance. The muscles along the spine are very powerful muscles, and if they remain tight and out of balance, they will begin pulling on the segments of the spine. This causes stress in the spinal anatomy, which can hinder the vertebrae's ability to move independently from each other.

This warping puts more pressure on the nerves; the nerves then begin to affect the muscles, and the muscles affect the bone. It is a bad cycle that spirals downward over time. It could take decades, but eventually the muscles and bones begin to break down and no longer function well. With chiropractic adjustments, you can break the cycle to improve health and well-being.

PHYSICAL STRESS

People experience multiple physical traumas throughout their lifetime: sports injuries, bike accidents, falling episodes, etc. Another large component of physical problems, especially in today's society, includes the type of activities—or lack of activity—we do regularly. Many people sit for eight hours at a time in front of a computer and then go home where they sit and watch television for several hours. A large portion of physical stress has to do with our current type of lifestyle and work environment. Car accidents, surgeries, and even bad mattresses are all stressors for the body.

The primary physical stressor is the actual birthing process, especially in the case of an assisted birth with forceps, because it causes stress and traction injuries on the newborn's spinal column and neck. The most dangerous journey you take in your life is through the birth canal. Multiple studies have shown that any type of forced delivery causes tremendous stress in the brain stem area (where the brain and spinal cord meet), causing all manner of illnesses in children: behavioral problems, failing to thrive, sleeping problems, bedwetting, etc. All of these things begin to develop because the child's neurology was damaged at birth.

EMOTIONAL STRESS

Of all stresses that I see in our office, emotional stress is the biggest one. It is also the most devastating of stresses; it has a profound impact on our neurology. People tend to worry by nature, and with the constant barrage of bad news from the media, it can be hard to ever stop worrying. People are designed to handle stress in isolated bursts—for example, a primitive man may have seen a poisonous snake, been alarmed, and calmed down when the threat was gone. People today, however, worry about their family, money, and the world constantly, and their stress hormones never have a chance to normalize. This leads to rapid aging and chronic diseases. These devastating stress-related health conditions are growing at an alarming rate.

CHEMICAL STRESS

From pharmaceutical drugs that we take for various conditions to foreign chemicals that appear in our water, we are surrounded by chemical stressors. Chemical stressors are in cigarette smoke, immunization shots (which can include mercury or formaldehyde), and the preservatives in our food. Some of us use artificial sweeteners that have a variety of unnatural chemicals. It is a long, long list. More than 10 years ago, the Red Cross did a study[1] using the blood of newborns taken from the umbilical cord. They discovered over 200 neurotoxins in this blood, showing that we are exposed to a toxic environment even before birth.

THE THREE DIVISIONS OF THE NEUROLOGICAL SYSTEM

Physiologists around the world have begun to realize that our health is a reflection of how we adapt to our environment. Our neurology provides adaptation for the body, and if a person cannot adapt to the surrounding environment, they will lose their health.

There are two parts of the neurological system. The first is the central nervous system, which consists of the brain and spinal cord. The second consists of the peripheral nerves, which branch out from the spinal cord to other areas of the body, providing a life force.

We also have three groups of nerves: sensory, motor, and autonomic. Our motor nerves tell our muscles how to function, our sensory nerves allow us to feel and experience our environment and the autonomic nerves control the functions we don't have to think about: organs, glands, blood vessels, and the organizing controls of the body. Our sensory nerves represent only 10 percent of the neurological system. That means that 90 percent of the nerves that provide the "life force" of the body have no pain fibers. These motor nerves, also referred to as functional nerves, can be damaged or disturbed without any apparent symptoms until the condition is at an advanced or life-threatening stage.

SPECIFIC CONDITIONS TREATED WITH CHIROPRACTIC

ADHD: In an increasing number of sensory deprivation cases, children cannot process the world normally, and so they shut down. These children develop ADHD, autism, or other neurologically-based disorders. While there are many theories on the reason this is happening, I believe that there are too many chemicals in a child's system at an early age, which has a negative impact on the child's neurological system. Children may not eat healthy foods, exercise, or receive any encouragement or love at home. They may also have excessive exposure to technology. All of these things can cause them to just shut down.

Chiropractic is just one of the many keys to helping a child suffering from spectrum disorders such as ADHD, which is a sensory problem. Chiropractors correct subluxations, which are interferences of the neurological network rooted in the three stressors mentioned earlier. Subluxations not only affect the physical body but can distort a person's perception of his or her world, preventing him or her from processing things correctly.

Our office uses specific chiropractic care in the brain stem area, which is in the upper part of the neck. In most cases, when a child comes to me with ADHD, I find a subluxation in the first two segments of the spine. Since the neurology is not functioning properly, the child cannot correctly process the world around him or her in all its complexity and constant change. Along with proper diet and exercise, chiropractic care can help the child to deal with his or her surrounding world, thereby reducing the rate of ADHD.

Physically, the child becomes more aware of his or her environment and starts to lose the frustration and anger. After chiropractic care, we have seen that children are better able to focus, concentrate, make eye contact, communicate, and sleep more soundly. Combined with a proper diet and exercise, we see huge improvements. It is truly a mystery to me how so few people can be aware of the lifestyle changes that need to happen to accomplish those improvements.

Personally, I have a great passion for taking care of children. Children are my favorite patients, and it is wonderful to see these kids turn around after proper treatment and care.

Arthritis: There are many different forms of arthritis. The problem is not the specific type of arthritis but the damage or decay that it inflicts on the spinal nerves. The purpose of the spinal column is to protect the spinal cord from injury, just as our skull protects our brain. Nature provides the necessary armor.

When a person begins to have decay or arthritis in the spine, a domino or "cascade" effect begins to negatively impact health in general. More pressure on the spinal nerves spreads throughout the body, reducing the blood and nerve supply, which leads to a lack of vitality. When a person has arthritis in the spine, the joints are stuck. If joints do not move, they begin to decay rather rapidly. Chiropractic care offers mobility for the joints.

Chiropractors identify the areas of subluxation, where the spine has begun to decay. They administer adjustments in that area to regain mobility, get the blood supply flowing, and stimulate neurology so that their patient can get back to living a normal life.

Allergies: Allergies are an immune system response to overstimulation. After the healthy tissues are assaulted by foreign invaders, the immune system does not know when to shut down. Out of the many reasons for the increasing occurrence of allergies, the main cause is environmental: too many chemicals are being introduced to our bodies.

For example, our food supplies have been damaged with pesticides and herbicides. Your immune system is nothing more than a mobile form of your neurological system, which is very delicate. This may explain why chiropractors are continually seeing increased numbers of patients with allergy problems.

Quite honestly, I believe that there are too many immunization shots for children. This is not healthy for their immune responses and is one reason we see allergies and asthma developing in children. When I was a child, there were four or five shots available. Now there are 60 to 70 immunity shots recommended to children before they reach the age of 18. Even though there's a lot of professional literature that supports the idea of limiting immunization shots, immunizations are a large industry, and their use has been ingrained in our society.

Pregnancy: Most chiropractic techniques are safe for a pregnant woman, and quite a few very gentle techniques are available for women in any stage of pregnancy. Chiropractic care involves much more than simply moving a bone from Point A to Point B. It is more about stimulating the neurology. In my career, I have met many pregnant women who did very well throughout their pregnancy with chiropractic care. It is quite safe for pregnant women.

Chronic Fatigue Syndrome: While our bodies produce energy every day through mitochondria (the powerhouses of our cells), if you are not living a healthy lifestyle and are overwhelmed with stressors, your body cannot function well. This will cause your neurology to shut down. Stressors hinder us from producing the energy we need so that our lack of neurological function results in fatigue rather than vitality.

As vital living beings, we produce energy every day—at a minimum, the body is designed to do that. If we are not making enough energy to get through a day, we tap into what we refer to as functional reserves, like a reserve tank in a luxury car. When you are routinely tapping into your functional reserves, it is exhaustive to your system, making you susceptible to chronic diseases.

We can measure a person's heart rate variability to determine the functional reserves, which are our vital force. When healthcare providers see patients with low heart rate variability who are tapping into the reserves, they wake up tired every day and are tired throughout the day. When I see patients who have this issue, I take the time to educate them, review their health concerns, and make the connection between their concerns and their heart rate variability. When they know that chiropractic care provides a solution that will relieve the fatigue, using some fascinating technology, the lights go on inside these patients. It is truly remarkable.

Obesity: Obesity is an epidemic, and it was recently shown to cause more health problems than smoking. Most people focus on calorie intake, which is very important, but research shows that there are multiple reasons for obesity, including lack of sleep. Researchers have also shown that emotional stress from a young age can increase a person's likelihood to be obese. Emotional stress actually has a bigger impact on obesity than calorie intake.

Of course, lifestyle choices have a huge impact on the rate of obesity in our country as well. People often sit all day at work, are sedentary at home, do not eat a healthy diet, and are stressed all the time. Naturally, they will gain weight.

Whiplash and Automobile Accidents: There is a lot of science behind the mechanisms of whiplash and its treatments, all based on physics. Dr. Arthur Croft at the Crash Institute of San Diego is the leading authority in the country on crash reenactments. He's shown that even a minor fender bender at eight miles per hour, or a low-impact car accident, can cause devastating damage to your neck, and you may not realize it until years later.

Whiplash injuries are devastating. Typically, following an accident, a person will go to the emergency room.. If the initial examination and x-rays show no fractures or hemorrhages, the patient is often instructed to go home, take pain pills, and call their doctor if there are continual problems. Years later, when these accident survivors visit my office, they have no idea that the long-ago automobile accident is causing them to experience problems now. However, they are often searching for a non-pharmaceutical solution because they haven't seen results with pain medication or they want to stop taking so much medicine.

In an accident, there might be multiple people in the same car; some may be seriously injured while others may show no signs of injury. This has a lot to do with the force that enters the body and position of the head. Sometimes, while reviewing the history of a new patient, I discover that the patient was in an automobile accident at some time in the past and that no corrective or follow-up procedures were performed. In most cases, the person will show decay in the spine and neck. He or she may show severe degeneration of the cervical spine. Generally, if an accident victim does not seek the proper care by a highly skilled chiropractor within the first six weeks, he or she has a 90 percent chance of experiencing neck pain off and on for the remainder of his or her life.

Proper chiropractic care for automobile accidents is about joint mobilization. Without mobilization, the vertebrae do not move independently from each other; they begin to break down, become inflamed, and can begin the decay process within the first six weeks. In an accident, your neck goes beyond its normal range. This causes ligaments to stretch or tear, tendons to rupture, muscles to become inflamed and scarred, and inflammation to set in, causing further destruction to the structures of the spine.

With a new patient, we do thorough orthopedic and neurological testing. One of the first tests we perform is orthopedic testing (Foraminal Compression) that checks for occlusions (narrowing) in the openings along the spinal column (vertebral foramens). These occlusions cause numbness and tingling in the arms or hands. The purpose of this test is to compress the neck vertebrae to assess whether or not the nerves are irritated enough to provoke shooting pains or numbness. We are extremely careful with this test because any compression can cause a lot of pain, although it won't cause more damage.

Another common procedure is a Davis series of five to seven x-rays: front view, mouth open, side view, flexion–extension, left oblique, and right oblique. These will show the nerve exits and whether or not the foramens have been damaged or occluded in any way. I'll usually suggest chiropractic treatment. However, if

I see considerable damage, we would then refer the patient to have an MRI scan to fully view the extent of the damage.

There are several variables to consider before determining the length of time needed for the patient to see improvement: age, overall health, severity of the injury, and date of the accident's occurrence. Even in severe cases, the average patient begins to see some improvement within eight to ten visits, though full spinal healing may take between 12 and 14 months. (For a reference point, it often takes years of braces on kids' teeth to accomplish a process of healing.) In mild cases, the patient begins to see improvement within two or three visits. In some cases, we see instant improvement when the patients say, "Wow, I can turn my head!"

BENEFITS OF CHIROPRACTIC CARE

Most of our patients come to the office focused on a specific problem that is their sole concern, such as headaches or back pain. They usually think that these are the only issues they can resolve in our office. They are amazed when I relate some of the side benefits of chiropractic care: better quality sleep, more energy throughout the day, more focus, more mental clarity, better digestion, reduced need for medications, increased range of motion, and a feeling of youth without medical side effects.

When a patient walks into my office, the first thing that he or she should understand is that I am not the healer. The body does the healing. I just remove the pressure from the neurology and work with the structure while providing tips to improve the person's lifestyle.

Neurology runs the body. It is the driving force that tells the body how to function. If there is damage or interference to the nerves that go to an organ, this organ (liver, stomach, lungs, heart, etc.) cannot function properly. The purpose of a chiropractic adjustment is to remove interference or disturbance from the neurological system so that it can send the proper messages to the target organ and begin to function as intended.

Our bodies are very adaptive. You may not be aware of an issue in your body because there are no symptoms until the condition has advanced beyond the point at which the body can adapt. When our body fails to adapt, it begins producing symptoms. For example, if you were to ask a person how he felt the day before his heart attack, he would probably say, "I felt fine." Obviously, something was seriously wrong, but symptoms didn't emerge until the actual heart attack.

We see this principle in chiropractic care. A person arrives at the office and says, "My neck started bothering me last week." When we perform tests and take x-rays, we see evidence of spinal decay going back 15 to 20 years or more with no apparent symptoms. If a person experiences a physical trauma (i.e., a serious fall, car accident, sporting accident, etc.), he or she should be checked by a chiropractor because there could be damage without symptoms.

NEW TECHNOLOGIES IN THE LAST DECADE

One of my favorite new technologies is called the INSiGHT™ Subluxation Station. It combines four different technologies on a single platform, one of which is referred to as a thermal scan. The human body is symmetrical by nature. Our left and right sides should basically be the same. Thermal scans have heat-sensitive cameras that examine a person's spine by looking at the left side and the right side of the spine. As the patient sits in a controlled environment with an even temperature, the scan reveals variations in bodily temperature from the left side and the right side and flags any temperature differences. This is significant because the autonomic nerve system, which represents 90 percent of our neurology, controls blood vessels that need to dilate and constrict to adapt to our environment. Temperature variations indicate with certainty that there are disturbances within that group of nerves. Since these are functional nerves and not sensory nerves, there are usually no symptoms. However, that area of the body is not functioning correctly because the neurology is demonstrating that it is disturbed or interfered with as evidenced by the temperature change.

We also use INSiGHT™ to test the range of motion of the cervical spine to find any restrictions. This is performed using an algometer. The range of motion needs to be equal on left and right sides; proper range of motion is essential to remain youthful. Motion is life.

Another part of the INSiGHT™ system is the Surface Electromyography (sEMG), which looks at the function of a type of nerve called a "motor nerve." There are trillions of motor nerves throughout the body providing functions for the muscles. When these nerves are not functioning correctly, muscles will become weak, tight, or spasmodic. Chiropractors look for imbalances in the muscles around the spine. When there are imbalances, the person will have pain as well as a lack of motion. They also fatigue easily because the body is not operating very efficiently. It's impossible for a body to operate efficiently while dealing with muscle imbalances. Usually, these patients also show achy joints, motion restrictions, and poor posture along with the fatigue.

Then we look at heart rate variability by looking at the nerves that control the function of the heart; when these nerves are out of balance, it predisposes a person to heart attack. The autonomic nervous system is broken into two parts, sympathetic and parasympathetic. As mentioned earlier, chiropractors need to ensure that their patients are not routinely tapping into their functional reserves.

We use these technologies together to arrive at the "core score" or the Neuro-Spinal Functional Index (NSFI). As the number increases, the health of the person increases. At the beginning, we get a base line to determine the patient's overall health and wellness. We perform a series of chiropractic adjustments (generally about ten to twelve) and then run the tests again. As we perform adjustments, we see the NSFI increase. Typically, the patient begins to see side benefits such as more energy, better sleep, and improved bodily functions.

It might seem like these four technologies would take a great deal of time to operate. However, since our office can assess all four of these areas at one time, the process doesn't take long. Typically, we perform all four on the first visit, which usually takes about 15 minutes, and then we get the NSFI core score. This allows us to more accurately discover the trouble spots in their neurology, so that we can practice with better skill and help people get well with more certainty.

CHIROPRACTIC TECHNIQUES

There are three main types of chiropractic techniques. The first is more of a structural approach where we move a bone from one area to another. The second is based on muscle techniques, and the third is based on the neurological approach. The neurological approach makes more sense to me because that is the master system of the body, helping the entire body to function and repair itself.

Our office uses a very specific, very gentle tonal technique for the neurological approach. It is a repeatable technique that is specific and low-force but produces wonderful results. Some chiropractors still use the high-force technique, but I have moved away from that with better results for my patients.

OUR HEALTHCARE SYSTEM

Our healthcare system (or "sick care" system) in this country is not very efficient, because it treats symptoms rather than promoting a healthy lifestyle. My colleague, Dr. Patrick Gentempo, said, "If you offer sick care to a population, you end up with sick people."

Even though insurance is based on sick care, most chiropractic care is covered by insurance policies. However, since insurance companies typically don't offer enough coverage for the long-term care a patient needs to really get well, our office is doing everything we can to get away from insurance because it's a losing game. Since 80% of our patients pay in cash, we're basically a cash practice at this point. Personally, I just don't believe that insurance companies exist to serve people, and I refuse to be a slave to these companies rather than serve my community with quality care.

Furthermore, the solutions offered by typical medical care are centered on taking prescription drugs which do not give a return on a person's quality of life; drugs only cover symptoms rather than treating the cause. The healthcare system has outstanding emergency care that is good at saving lives, but it does not have effective answers for chronic problems or illnesses. There are very few medical solutions meant to address those things that prevent a person from living a healthy life.

The chiropractic principles never change, since they are based on biological laws and universal principles. What will change is the social perception of chiropractic care. My biggest professional enemy is a basic misunderstanding about what is offered by chiropractic care. Most people think that it is only a neck and back "thing," but it offers so much more than that because it's based on wellness.

The beautiful thing about chiropractic care is that it is proactive rather than waiting until there are symptoms of sickness. Chiropractic care finds the cause and then allows the natural healing of the body to do its job. Despite heavy opposition, chiropractors have been preaching this message from the rooftops for 119 years: lifestyle, healthy choices, proper exercise, proper diet, proper rest, and stress management. Chiropractic care helps a person's neurology to achieve balance and stimulates that neurology to make a healthier person.

By contrast, the medical system is just about bankrupt. The amount of gross domestic product spent on healthcare (18 percent) is staggering . Not long ago, I saw an interview with a few retired military officers, a general, and an admiral. They said that our country is entering a crisis because it's so difficult to find healthy young people to serve in the military. A country must have healthy people in order to have a robust military for protection. The message of chiropractic care is based on wellness, which is the future of healthcare. My best patients are the ones who have no symptoms but come in regularly for care so they can live up to their potential.

When you receive chiropractic care routinely, it increases your ability to adapt to the stresses of the world. The best example I can give would be an Army Ranger or Navy Seal. They endure so much physical and emotional stress that very few can go through the whole program without breaking down. The ones who make it through are the healthiest people on the planet because they have the widest gap of adapting.

Your nervous system is your master system, controlling, coordinating, and adapting to the environment. If you interfere with this system, you interfere with function and quality of life. There is no condition that would disqualify a person from chiropractic care because with a higher functioning nervous system, you have a greater chance of recovering from any health problem.

When you receive routine chiropractic care, it widens your gap of adapting to the stresses of the world. It improves immune function so that all bodily systems can work better. Chiropractic care is a very powerful way to naturally and safely maintain and increase your health and is designed for people who are wellness-minded.

(This content should be used for informational purposes only. It does not create a doctor-patient relationship with any reader and should not be construed as medical advice. If you need medical advice, please contact a doctor in your community who can assess the specifics of your situation.)

References:

[1]"Body Burden: The Pollution In Newborns." *Environmental Working Group*, 14 Jul. 2005. http://www.ewg.org/research/body-burden-pollution-newborns.

3

A Rare,
Generational
Perspective

by Daniel Grossman D.C.

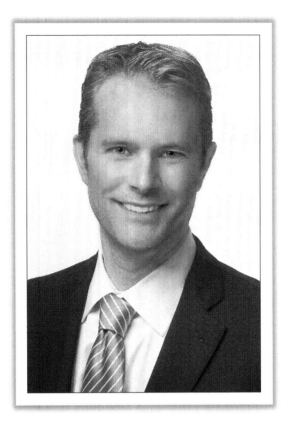

Daniel Grossman D.C.
Generations Physical Medicine
Middletown, New Jersey
www.njspinecare.com

Dr. Daniel Grossman is a third-generation chiropractor. He has treated thousands of patients, including high profile professional athletes, entertainers, executives, physicians, and members of the community. He is a cum laude graduate of the Los Angeles College of Chiropractic and has been practicing in New Jersey since 1997.

Dr. Grossman is a past NY/NJ Course Chairman of the Los Angeles College of Chiropractic ACRB Diplomat in Rehabilitation program 1997-2001. He is a Fellow of the American Board of Disability Analysts. He is a certified McKenzie and Cox Distraction practitioner. He is certified in Manipulation under Anesthesia. He has been qualified by the Superior Courts of New York and New Jersey as an Expert in Chiropractic. He serves as a chiropractic and ergonomic consultant to numerous large companies and institutions. He has extensive experience in Non-Surgical Spinal Decompression, MUA, and chiropractic rehabilitation.

A RARE, GENERATIONAL PERSPECTIVE

I was literally born into the world of chiropractic care. When my mother went into labor, my father had to leave his patients in the clinic to attend my birth. To this day, I still don't think it was a good enough excuse to leave the office early.

Our family, beginning with my grandfather (who established his chiropractic roots back in the 1930s), founded the very practice in which I work today. I'm a third-generation chiropractor, one of 15 chiropractors to come from one of the oldest chiropractic families in the world today.

My family first practiced in 1930. In that year, Herbert Hoover was the president, Pluto was discovered, and the chocolate chip cookie was first created. I'm fortunate to treat patients in a practice that has been going strong since 1941. In fact, our practice was started the same year as NBC and CBS. Franklin Delano Roosevelt was president of the United States, the world was in the grip of WWII, and Bugs Bunny made his debut. Yes, we are as old as Elmer Fudd

Our family history and longevity give our practice some truly unique advantages. Some patients have been treated by our family for generations. One patient, now age 104, has been a regular patient for 70 years. She started coming here as a young lady in her 30s; she was treated by my family before her children, who are now in their late 70s (and are also patients), were born.

This ability to access the gamut of ups and downs in the life history of a patient—medical and otherwise—provides us with a unique and unprecedented perspective. We have the privilege of establishing a position of trust and respect that can only come with time and experience. Also, the tangible and intangible benefits reach beyond the personal knowledge that we have about our patients.

Treating multiple members of the same family provides a truly unique lens through which to view their medical issues; we can help patients more effectively by seeing similarities in their anatomical conditions. Treating multiple members of the same family over decades shows an even more amazing, panoramic view of what makes them who they are. Other doctors can only dream about this remarkable vista. We can look at today's symptom and know that it is part of a family pattern or begin to see commonalities from generation to generation. Not only can we better treat them today, we can also anticipate and prepare for problems down the road. It's a profound perspective, allowing us to step back and see patterns that may otherwise go unnoticed.

The other advantage of growing up in this practice is the fact that I view these patients as my extended family. When I evaluate a problem or receive requests for help, I make the same recommendations and provide the same level of care that I would provide my immediate family. I trust that physicians always try to do the best they can in a fifteen-minute appointment, but when you see a person year after year for decades, you have a relationship with a firmer foundation and a more developed level of communication. The more relevant guidance stems from your more intimate understanding of that patient.

IT'S ALL ABOUT YOU

Traditional medicine and chiropractic care really have the same goal: the optimal health and well-being of the patient. Our approach to patient care, however, can prove to be vastly different.

In the dogmatic medical model, a patient goes to the physician and describes the symptoms. The physician evaluates the patient, orders appropriate testing, then prescribes medicine. The patient is often advised to return only if the symptoms do not resolve. A patient might have questions for the doctor, but essentially the conversation is a one-way street: Doctors order, patients comply.

In contrast, the chiropractic model has always has been aimed at the empowerment of the patient. Our goal is to keep the patient involved in his or her own care from the very beginning. Our discipline has always encouraged patients to ask questions about their conditions and to help themselves by observing and remaining active in their own care. As chiropractors, we tend to view our role as something of a conduit to enable the patients to heal themselves, finding ideal health and balance through a combination of passive care and active lifestyle changes.

In today's evolving healthcare arena, this perspective has stood the test of time. With the advent of Google and social media, and the sudden availability of information at our fingertips, many patients come in to the office after having done serious research already. They have many questions and come to us with very good, educated, and engaging discussion points about their condition and about their options. From a chiropractic perspective, it's a wonderful and essential conversation to have, a two-way street that traditional medicine is just starting to appreciate. Chiropractic has been embracing this for a century, because our goals are always to educate and empower our patients as much as possible, as they take a strong, productive and proactive role in their health.

The chiropractic profession continues to have one of the strongest satisfaction rates among any healthcare provider. While Western medicine is more symptom-driven, from early on, chiropractors have treated the patient, not just the symptoms. The injury or disease that patients present with doesn't exist in a vacuum. Their diet, overall health, current life situation, occupation, and psychosocial considerations all have a bearing on their current condition. These components of their lives may move the scale one way or another, and should never be ignored.

Our practice likes to take a very comprehensive and thoroughly proactive approach in providing patients with the proper treatment and lifestyle modifications, by including both active and passive intervention. Through chiropractic care, physical therapy, and at times pharmacologic intervention, we enable patients to achieve a level that they never thought possible. We measure success not only in reduction of pain and symptoms, but more importantly, in return to function and, ultimately, achievement of optimal outcomes. Success for one patient might involve completing a marathon, whereas success for another patient might involve simply walking a block.

UNDERSTANDING PAIN

The source of any and all pain in the body can be put into one of three categories:

a) Chemical

b) Mechanical

c) Emotional

Chemical pain includes those physiologic conditions that affect cellular metabolism and blood supply. Inflammation and ischemia are included in this category. Some painful conditions with a chemical origin include Rheumatoid Arthritis, Cancer, Lyme disease, bronchitis, and psoriasis. Acute injuries can also fall into this category. For example, if you whack your thumb with a hammer, the immediate pain you feel is primarily chemical due to acute inflammation. The secondary pain would be, of course, from embarrassment.

Mechanical pain includes any damage to the structure of tissue. Examples of mechanical pain can include disc herniation, broken bone, nerve compression (sciatica), subluxation, ligament sprain, and degenerative arthritis. The majority of chiropractic treatment strategy focuses on this category. Chiropractors are biomechanical experts.

In contrast, the majority of traditional (non-surgical) medicine falls into the chemical treatment strategy. Medicine is prescribed to address and alter the chemical and physiologic processes in the body. Medical doctors are pharmacologic experts.

Emotional/psychogenic pain includes any disorder that may be caused by, or exacerbated by, emotional or behavioral factors. Doctor John Sarno published a very compelling book some years ago: *Healing Back Pain, the Mind and Body Connection*. He describes a condition he calls tension myositis syndrome (TMS), in which he contends that the vast majority of chronic pain syndromes can be traced to an emotional component. That doesn't discount the pain as "all in your head," by any means. The pain is very real. Nevertheless, it comes from one of those three pain sources and emotional pain could be a factor. I always tell patients that the same brain that controls your heartbeat also controls your heart.

Given this fact, it follows that for anybody who comes in suffering with pain, there's almost always some component of each of the three pain sources. For example, a patient comes in with acute low back pain, which is also radiating down his leg. We examine the patient, send out for diagnostic testing, and determine that the patient has a disc herniation. In this case, the patient's disc herniation is a mechanical form of pain, which is compressing on a nerve. That compression causes inflammation, which also is contributing to his pain in a chemical way. When we dig a little deeper, we find out the patient is currently in the middle of a nasty divorce. The pain in the back has recently become more severe due to the emotional component.

As chiropractors, we take great care to address all these sources of pain. Chiropractors are experts in the mechanical side of treatment through adjustments and other treatments. In the office, we can mechanically address the problem by aligning vertebrae, reducing muscle spasm, increasing the space between joints, and reducing compression on the nerves. The chemical side, the inflammation, can be addressed through different modalities that we perform in the office: ultrasound, cold laser, various manipulative techniques, or just ice to reduce the inflammation. In some situations, though, the chemical side of pain needs to be mitigated through medication.

It works very nicely to have a combination of remedies (including the pharmacological remedy) to augment the active mechanical side of the equation, which is the chiropractic specialty. The emotional component can often be handled well by virtue of the relationship that we actively maintain with our patients. Those relationships—particularly if they are long-term—can help the patient deal with some of that emotional upheaval and the stressors that may be contributing to the acute flare-up. As such, chiropractors can, and do, exercise a large influence on all three components of the pain equation. We find that a combination of the mechanical and the chemical can make a profound impact on how a patient responds to treatment and care.

Successful and effective treatment strategies must be based on the nature of the condition. Sometimes only medicine will bring down severe inflammation. Sometimes only an adjustment will restore normal motion to a joint, eliminating pain. The best physicians will identify the condition and recognize which categories apply. They will then treat, co-manage, or refer as appropriate.

CHIROPRACTIC AN UNDERSUNG SCIENCE

I often hear the phrase, "I believe in chiropractic." While I appreciate the tone and spirit of the expression, I disagree with the core philosophy. While "belief" supports confidence and trust, it also suggests a faith based ideology. You don't often hear people saying, "I believe in dentistry." It's pretty much a given that if you value your teeth, you will ascribe to the benefits of dentistry.

Chiropractic, like dentistry, is, in fact, not a belief; it is a science, a philosophy, and an art. The science is well published. The extensive research and articles contained in textbooks and journals are from the leading institutions in the world. The federal government (Medicare) and the insurance industry simply would not cover any procedure or treatment they deem not to be scientifically sound or worthy of inclusion. Chiropractic is the third largest profession of healthcare delivery in the world behind traditional medicine and dentistry.

The core philosophy of chiropractic is that chiropractic manipulation positively affects both the central nervous system and musculoskeletal systems. While we put an emphasis on the mechanical component of disease management, we are sure to incorporate the chemical and emotional sources in effectively treating patients.

The art of diagnosing and adjusting comes with time, skill, and lots of practice. Like dentistry, you know when you've been to an excellent chiropractor. The difference between techniques and skill level can be profound. If you are not reaching your goals with treatment, consider trying a physician with a different technique or skill set.

Chiropractors, like all physicians, do not heal you. In fact, there has never been a doctor in existence who could heal any patient. It is only the patient that has the ability to heal. The physician's role is to provide a stimulus to facilitate the innate healing process. The difference lies in the tools used to provide this stimulus: chiropractors adjust, medical doctors prescribe, surgeons cut.

THE PERFECT CHIROPRACTIC PATIENT

If you possess a spine, you're off to a good start. Beyond that, there's really no typical chiropractic patient. Rather, our practice represents a cross section of life--a smorgasbord of humanity with the common goal of optimal health. We treat children, elderly patients, doctors, lawyers, priests, and nuns. We treat construction workers, mail carriers, and stay at home moms. We treat elite, highly functioning professional athletes and patients with physical disabilities, as well as everybody clustered somewhere in the middle. Some days our waiting room is like a Woody Allen movie. Have you ever seen a 4'10", 102 lb. grandmother sitting next to a 6'7", 380 lb. lineman?

This variety of patients gives us a tremendous appreciation for the differences in human beings and, best of all, gives us the opportunity to positively affect a comprehensive array of people on many different levels.

The goal for one patient may be completely different from the objectives of another patient. For example, one person may come in with the relatively simple goal of getting rid of the acute pain that's radiating down her leg. Another patient may arrive, saying, "I'm looking to improve my function so I can take four strokes off my golf game."

Other patients may come in seeking a complete lifestyle change. From them, we hear, "I've been dealing with chronic pain for many years. I'm overweight and I want to make a change. I'm fed up with the pain. I want to adopt a completely different lifestyle and a different set of habits towards optimal health." Those are the patients with whom we can work very closely over a period of time to help them and, essentially, transform their lives. The applicability of chiropractic care is very profound; it can, based on the patient's needs and goals, truly change their lives.

That is one of the most rewarding things that I have found in my practice: just seeing these amazing transformations of our patients.

We see them come in suffering with pain, or awash in a sense of defeat, because the long-term pain and dysfunction have wrung the very life out of them. Later, to see such a profound change in them is incredibly rewarding. We're fortunate to see how our treatments can affect their attitude, their ability to function, and the difference in quality of life for them and their families. More often than not, it is the spouse, the significant other, or another family member of the patient who will come in and tell me how much better that person is feeling. Often, patients will say, "I'm doing much better," but the full extent of their improvement is usually best viewed through the eyes of their family. Those are the folks who see, on a daily basis, the incredible change that the treatments brought about. It's so rewarding when a mother or a wife will come in and say, "Thank you for giving my Lauren her life back," or, "Thank you for giving Brandon the ability to work and to support our family again." It just doesn't get much better than that.

This is the reason I wake up every day and come to work. Even after spending a lifetime in chiropractic, I'm still overcome by the joy of helping my patients. We've always assumed and expected that our patients will get well. We set a very high standard for ourselves and for them. We expect that they are going to achieve the goals we've set together. Only very rarely do we find that those goals seem difficult or impossible. When such a situation presents itself, we will often explore a variety of different options and recruit a multidisciplinary team to assure we leave no stone unturned. Ultimately, we find the right combination that works for each patient.

So there is no "standard procedure," nor is there a cookie-cutter approach to a patient. Every person who comes to us is different. Each person we see brings to us different needs, different goals, and a totally different set of circumstances. And a spine.

THE CHIROPRACTIC JOURNEY

In the early 1900s, the Palmer family, who are truly the first family of chiropractic care, founded the Palmer School of Chiropractic and weren't taken very seriously. In those days, chiropractic care was viewed skeptically. The medical community did not generally accept chiropractic theory. Starting with one college in Davenport, Iowa (The Palmer School), it was a matter of proving our worth over time. In the early days, the medical profession had an adversarial relationship with chiropractic. Not only was our discipline a source of competition, it represented the first formally organized alternative to mainstream medicine. In the early days of unquestioned medical dogma, this challenge to the conventional wisdom of medicine was simply unheard of.

My grandfather started his practice in a day when there was quite a bit of resistance. However, in time, and with such indisputable results, chiropractic care began to prove itself as a valid companion piece to traditional medicine. The field gained steam over the years. Eventually, the patients' demand for chiropractic treatment essentially legitimized the field. This took place at about the time my father was practicing in the 1970s and 1980s. There came a transitional period, during which doctors began to open their eyes a little and see some benefit in what we do. Those MDs started to refer patients sparingly— very sparingly at first—to chiropractors. In this practice, we've always been very fortunate to have excellent working relationships with many primary care physicians, medical doctors and specialists in the community for over half a century.

In 1972, Medicare finally approved chiropractic care as a covered benefit. From that point until now, most major insurance carriers have come to accept chiropractic as a viable and preferred treatment option. That was the turning point—the point at which chiropractic became mainstream and began to enjoy broader acceptance.. Chiropractic has proven, time after time, to deliver superior results at a fraction of the cost of medicine and surgery. Insurance companies recognize this, and as a result, also benefit from chiropractic's value.

Today, most especially in our state, there is growing integration within the medical and chiropractic communities.

In my practice, there are medical doctors, physical therapists, acupuncturists, and even orthopedic and neurosurgeons working together to meet the needs of our patients. This collaboration offers the opportunity to enjoy a fruitful symbiotic relationship, in which we can best help our patients achieve optimal results.

Chiropractic has come a long way. Our profession has evolved to not only remain relevant, but also lead healthcare towards the emerging trend of progressive, yet conservative, care. There's unprecedented cooperation, collaboration, and mutual respect between the medical and chiropractic professions, now that there's a better understanding of exactly what we do and of our role in the broader healthcare picture.

PROGRESS TOWARD OPTIMAL HEALTH

I think that the advantage of having a practice that's been around for 75 years is that it truly provides the broad picture perspective: issues become so much more apparent in treatment when you can see and analyze those things from our vantage point. Now that our profession is finally considered mainstream, I hope that more practices will have the kind of longevity that we're lucky and blessed to have here. As I look at the family history of a patient that we've been treating, whose mother and grandmother we treated, I have a much better understanding of their conditions and how to best help her.

Going forward, chiropractic's role in the healthcare of the future is very well-placed. On a larger healthcare framework, chiropractors really fill a very important role. Eighty-five percent of all people in the US will be disabled by an episode of back pain at some point in their lives. The total number of chiropractic office visits in the United States each year is 250 million, with 94% of all spinal manipulations performed by chiropractors. Back pain is the most frequent and expensive health care problem, and most common cause of work loss and disability among adults aged 30-50. Management and treatment of back pain has always been a fundamental role of chiropractic, so it stands to reason that chiropractors will remain at the forefront in public health efforts to effectively manage this epidemic.

For a long time chiropractors, especially in more rural areas, have actually functioned as primary care doctors or as the primary physician of the patient and family. Over time, we have been extremely fortunate to have been entrusted with that position of confidence by our patients. As health care continues to evolve, the trend is moving toward larger and more consolidated groups, and chiropractic care has a unique place in that model. As professionals, chiropractors bring a unique skill set and capacity for tremendous influence on patient behaviors. This makes us extremely helpful to patients, as we have a proactive hand in guiding their care on numerous levels. Further, research has proven that we can play an important and effective role in managing and treating not just spinal conditions, but a multitude of conditions such as diabetes, asthma, hypertension, premenstrual syndrome, infantile colic, vertigo, and obesity.

As healthcare moves forward, the trend will be towards less personal, more Eurocratic care: an approach similar to socialized medicine. While this may lead to greater efficiency, it will undoubtedly reduce the interpersonal nature of the doctor- patient relationship. Chiropractors, on the other hand, have always fostered strong personal relationships with our patients, providing a unique ability to shepherd the whole of their care. Chiropractors will prove to be influential in offering insightful guidance patients may otherwise not find in other forms of healthcare.

THERE'S ONLY ONE WAY TO TREAT A PATIENT

With respect.

THERE'S MORE THAN ONE WAY TO TREAT A BACK

In my opinion, the best chiropractors will have an assortment of techniques and technology in their chiropractic tool kits to offer patients throughout their course of care. When a patient initially comes to us, we examine and evaluate the condition through various means: reviewing the patient's health history, performing a clinical examination, ordering and performing the appropriate diagnostic tests, including, but not limited to, X-ray, MRI, CT, EMG/NCV, and blood tests. We then collect this data, sit down with the patient, and review in detail our findings. We will always offer multiple treatment options.

Most patients do very well with basic chiropractic and physical therapy intervention. This may include various chiropractic adjustments and techniques, stretching and strengthening exercises, electric muscle stimulation, cold laser, ultrasound, traction, etc. Patients are given a plan of treatment and scheduled for a re-evaluation to assess progress.

For more complicated cases we offer an array of services to significantly improve patient outcomes.

For disc herniations, one of the most powerful and effective treatments that I have seen is non-surgical spinal decompression. A disc herniation amounts to compression on a nerve. Ultimately, there are really only two ways you can relieve that compression: surgically or non-surgically.

With some rare exceptions, it is almost always preferential to treat discs non-surgically. In my experience, our non-surgical spinal decompression protocol has a very high success rate for a vast majority of people specifically suffering from disc

71

related symptoms. Utilizing a machine the size of an MRI unit, non-surgical decompression enables us to isolate the disc herniation, administer a force that effectively reduces the pressure inside the disc, and subsequently reduce or eliminate the disc's pressure on the spinal nerve roots. Non-surgical decompression creates a vacuum-like effect, pulling the disc off the nerve and relieving the patient's pain. This technique has proven to be one of the most effective treatments we offer, inclusive of surgery.

Another technique that offers profound results is called manipulation under anesthesia. In certain cases, we are unable to fully achieve our treatment goals. Some patients show a limited response in the clinical office setting due to pain, muscle guarding, pain-related resistance, or other motion-restricted conditions like a frozen shoulder or hip bursitis. In these cases, our anesthesiologist administers a twilight anesthesia in our outpatient surgery center, allowing us to painlessly treat the patient without the reflexive muscle guarding and spasm associated with these conditions. It also enables us to gently release scar tissue and adhesions surrounding the joint without pain. This incredibly useful technique can be implemented in very difficult cases and is often the "game changer" in long-term chronic pain situations that haven't been responsive to more traditional treatments. Patients suffering from degenerative arthritis, degenerative disc disease, fibromyalgia, myofascitis, adhesive capsulitis, bursitis, and other range of motion-limiting conditions may find tremendous improvement with this treatment.

We can also use a combination of chiropractic and interventional medical procedures to help reduce inflammation and restore function to the spine and joints. For example, we perform a technique called manipulation under joint anesthesia, which basically is a combination of manipulation under anesthesia and either a large joint injection, or a lumbar facet block. This procedure allows us to address the biomechanical joint dysfunction through manipulation, as well as the acute inflammation through introduction of a corticosteroid into the joint(s). This procedure is also performed under twilight sedation, and is a true collaboration between medical and chiropractic disciplines. The patient response is tremendous, and represents some of the best available techniques in one procedure.

One of the first goals in our practice is to gain a solid understanding of the types of treatments that our patients have already experienced. After learning what has worked and what may not have worked, we are able to then customize the treatment plan for that patient based on his or her specific needs. It's absolutely essential to pick a good chiropractor— someone who uses a variety of techniques and procedures—to help those cases that may be less responsive to basic chiropractic care.

THE "S" WORD

There can be a noticeable gap in philosophy between chiropractic care and some branches of traditional medical care. That gap generally occurs at the intersection of surgery and non-invasive treatment. The foundation of chiropractic has always emphasized care without the use of medicine or surgery. While chiropractic continues to provide tremendous relief for millions of people, no specialty can prove to be all things to all people. There is a time and place for medicine and surgery.

Keeping that in mind, I caution patients who may feel that surgery will be a panacea to their chronic problems. They imagine that there is some kind of guarantee associated with the procedure. Of course, there are no guarantees in life. I only advise surgical consultation if all reasonable conservative efforts fail. Statistically, that happens about 1% of the time.

In fact, a May 2013 article published in Spine found that patients who first consulted with a surgeon for their spinal condition had surgery 42.7% of the time. Patients who first consulted with a chiropractor had surgery 1.5% of the time. Certain cases, such as cauda equine syndrome, are absolute surgical necessities. The vast majority of the rest will overwhelmingly respond to conservative care, including chiropractic.

CHOOSING YOUR CHIROPRACTOR

One of the challenges of the chiropractic profession is that while there is a universal standard of care, there is no standard of technique. Different chiropractors have different styles, skills, and approaches to care. Some chiropractors may adjust the whole spine, others may just adjust one part of the spine (the upper cervical or first vertebrae, for example). Some adjust extremities, such as shoulders, hips, and knees. Others don't adjust at all, but rather utilize a device such as an activator to treat. Some patients do very well with the activator method. Others may feel this approach does not provide a "true" chiropractic adjustment.

This variety of techniques and care philosophy benefits patients in offering a wide array of options for various conditions. Conversely, it poses a challenge in continuity of care. For example, if you go to a dentist for the first time and don't receive the care you expected, you simply find another dentist. If a patient goes to a chiropractor for the first time and doesn't get the result they expected, they are more likely to feel that chiropractic as a whole did not help them. They'll comment "My husband tried chiropractic and it didn't help him." I'll ask "Did he try another chiropractor?" I usually get a blank stare. It just doesn't occur to them that, like going to an ineffective physician, they should simply find another one.

The technique and treatment style that works best for you may not work best for others. Therefore, it is very important as a patient to seek a physician who is skilled in various techniques, offers an array of modalities and treatment options, and has the ability and willingness to refer you to specialists if necessary. Most importantly, it MUST be someone with whom you feel comfortable, someone in whom you can confide, and someone with whom you can easily talk things over. You're looking for someone who can partner with you in helping you to achieve your healthcare goals. Again, in my opinion, the strongest role a chiropractor can play is helping and treating the entire patient—treating the whole person versus just treating the condition.

Chiropractic practitioners, like golfers, have multiple considerations to bring to their immediate "game." There's the hard science—the biomechanics, physiology, physics, the parameters of diagnosis—of evaluating the patient and identifying the condition; however, there is also a sizeable, profound art to the profession. The best golfers have an innate ability to read the situation. They then have the skill-set necessary to nail the swing. Chiropractic is very similar. It is important to find a chiropractor who has a very good innate ability to basically "read" the entire situation by accurately diagnosing the patient, effectively treating the patient, offering a comfortable technique, and having an amiable demeanor. This process includes so much more than just identifying the nature of the condition. A good practitioner looks at all facets of the patient's lifestyle, his job requirements, and certain psychosocial factors that could be contributing to the problem. It's a skill that takes years and thousands of patients to master.

If you are looking for a new chiropractor, I would recommend a two-pronged approach. First, ask around. Talk to family and friends and ask them who they go to. Pay attention to those who speak passionately about their doctor. It's always more compelling to speak with someone for whom a chiropractor has made a profound impact. "You have to go to Dr. Silverberg--he changed my life." "I crawled in to Dr. Grossman's office and walked out."

Second, consult your state's chiropractic association for a referral list. In New Jersey, our association is the ANJC (Association of New Jersey Chiropractors). They will usually have a phone number or website where you can research chiropractors by location, experience, training, etc.

Don't be limited by simply looking in your insurance provider book for a referral. Many top chiropractors elect to opt out of participation with certain insurance companies for a variety of reasons. The most common reason usually involves disagreements over patient care. Some plans significantly restrict care, or worse, try to dictate to the doctor how to treat a patient they've never met, let alone examined. Many doctors will simply not tolerate protocols they feel to be substandard or not beneficial to the patient.

A good chiropractor is worth his/her weight in gold.

A good chiropractor can literally change your life. Successful chiropractic care is a two-way street. I encourage you to follow up routinely with your doctor and always have objectives and goals for care. Help your chiropractor help you by keeping your communication open and honest. Be sure to do your part by following his advice and keeping your appointments. We can only help you if we see you.

(This content should be used for informational purposes only. It does not create a doctor-patient relationship with any reader and should not be construed as medical advice. If you need medical advice, please contact a doctor in your community who can assess the specifics of your situation.)

4

HEALING BY HAND

by Puneet Arora, D.C.

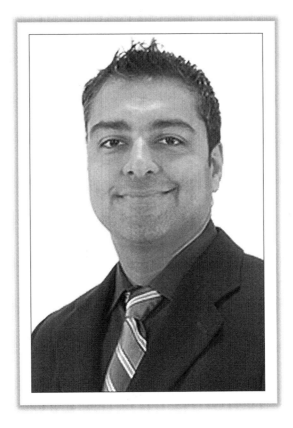

Puneet Arora, D.C.
Arora Family Chiropractic
Frisco, Texas
www.frisco-chiropractor.com

Dr. Puneet Arora received his Bachelor of Science undergraduate degree from the University of Toronto in 1997. In 2005, he earned his Doctor of Chiropractic degree from Northwestern Health Sciences University in Minneapolis, Minnesota. As he was wrapping up his studies in Minneapolis, he moved to Dallas to complete an externship and instantly fell in love with the Dallas/Fort Worth community and decided to settle there.

Dr. Arora's goal is to treat the patient as a whole by restoring optimum nervous system function and allowing the body to heal itself. As he states, time and time again, "I am not healing you, your body is healing itself. I'm just giving your body the push it needs in the right direction. Pain is just your body's way of letting you know something is wrong, much like the check engine light in your car. You can choose to ignore certain signals or like your car, get it checked out and find out what is really wrong."

HEALING BY HAND

I would like to shed light on the practice of Chiropractic and how our profession involves the concept of healing by hand. I find Chiropractic to be a rewarding occupation and look forward to each day in my element. Our practice focuses on healing patients and ultimately improving their quality of life. I often boast that because I have a self-fulfilling job, I LOVE Monday mornings and look forward to the start of another week of helping people. From our patient care to our community involvement, we actively participate in improving patient wellness.

One of our primary focal points is taking care of the "backbone" of families: the MOMS. Our four practices are very family-oriented. We believe that if you take care of the MOM, everything falls into place naturally. There is an old saying that we believe to be true: "When Mom is happy, everybody is happy." Since the mother in the family is usually the primary health care decision-maker and caregiver of the entire family, it is important that we start from the foundation and work from there.

Women come in for any number of reasons in the beginning, and when they see that we are able to offer affordable, non-surgical solutions that may resolve many health care issues, they begin to see us as their wellness "go-to" guys. We demonstrate how to assess and treat medical problems as naturally as possible. Women appreciate that our goal is to treat more than just the symptoms. In due time, we see Mom bring her high-school athlete and her sixth-grade daughter who has developed "text-neck" (more about that later), or a husband with a bad back who's been complaining for years without taking action. Usually, we see Moms getting frustrated with family members putting off treatment for various health issues which had been unresolved and have these family members accompany them to office visits so they can seek possible appropriate treatment. When we identify the problem and propose a solution, they immediately see the logic and expediency of our program. Eventually, families of three to five people are receiving treatment simultaneously when there is that initial recognition of the benefits of our care.

Moms are our biggest cheerleaders so we take very good care of them. In order to stay at the top of our patients' minds, it's important for us to be visible in the community. We stand on the sidelines of high school football games and we volunteer our time and energy for community events because our practices are geared toward families and communities. When you strive to be a good citizen and remain visible to the people who make up your community, ultimately you can take your place as a productive member. This isn't a sales gimmick—it's actually about giving back. When we give back, we get rewarded tenfold. Our rewards come in so many meaningful ways, not the least of which is helping people learn how to maintain their health.

CHIROPRACTIC EDUCATION

The education that a chiropractor must undertake is very similar to other doctors' medical education. Our education starts with a four-year undergraduate degree, followed by a post-graduate education (doctorate), which is typically a four-year program. A big focus of chiropractic education is hands-on experience and is a critical component of our training.

The last part of an education in chiropractic school, probably most of the final year, is hands-on clinical experience. We receive some training in the school setting, but for the most part, the last trimester is spent in an externship environment. As a student, you are paired up with a doctor who is willing to bring you on board and show you the true life experience of running a practice.

As far as certification is concerned, there are governing boards for every state. You must initially pass the national board exam, in addition to the respective state test. In the state of Texas, the licensing exam is called the Texas Jurisprudence Test. The successful completion of the aforesaid is necessary to commence Chiropractic practice.

We now participate as Mentor doctors in the internship/externship program. We sometimes get to spend three to six months with these new doctors as they are moving toward being full-fledged doctors of chiropractic care. That final phase includes not only patient care and the education of our patients on what we do, but it also includes instruction on other fundamental processes of the practice like documentation, billing, and integration with the community.

When we bring new doctors into our practice and help them to stand on their own feet, we also help to get them started in the community and teach them about giving back. That's the best part of chiropractic care, though they don't necessarily teach it or stress it in school: we do what we can to help our neighbors and the families around us. Not only does giving back make us a part of the community, we feel it is right thing to do from both a business and humanitarian perspective.

Involvement is a big thing that we stress with our younger doctors as well. We want them to adopt the same ideals and give back to the community as we do. Our goal in our work with junior doctors is that we can eventually partner with them and guide them through starting their own practice. We've been doing this for the last three or four years, and the program is working very well for us.

EDUCATION FOR OUR PATIENTS

In the beginning, many of our patients don't understand the exact nature of chiropractic care. Our first goal in treating a new patient is to educate him or her. Often, our patients come to us with a list of symptoms, usually neuro-musculoskeletal in nature. The symptoms could include subjective complaints such as back pain, persistent headaches, or even bursitis. When we are able to educate a new patient about the cause of the pain or "dis-ease", with help from a few diagnostic tests, we begin to narrow down the root of the problem. Then we propose possible solutions regarding treatment. This process helps us to objectify the subjective complaints.

At this point, we discuss insurance with our patients, which can be the most frustrating part of staying healthy. We take extra time to explain how our care fits into their insurance program, including the kinds of treatments that will and won't be covered by their insurance policy. Giving the patient the information that she needs to make an educated choice is usually appreciated in a big way and gives the patient a sense of empowerment. We don't use sales tactics or push the patient into a decision that she is not comfortable with. Once the patient is educated on options, we step back and let the patient decide how he or she wants to proceed. This may be a different approach compared to the realm of other healthcare practices because we want each patient to feel good about what we do and how we do it.

A NATURAL APPROACH

When people think of chiropractic medicine, they often think that it's all about the spine, though many patients also come in with headaches, allergies, and asthma. We deal primarily with the spine, because it is critically important, and taking the root pressure off of the nerves often helps deal with referred pain in the extremities.

Your spine is the highway your brain uses to communicate with all the rest of your body parts. The spine is flexible—or should be. If the spine were encased in a rod of steel, it wouldn't be as efficient because we wouldn't be able to twist and turn and bend. If the spinal vertebrae get subluxated (kinked out of alignment)— the spine doesn't move well and the entire operation (you and your body) can suffer from pinched nerves.

Given the opportunity, the body will heal itself in time. Sometimes, though, the body needs a gentle push in the right direction. With chiropractic manipulation, we help the body to work as it was designed to do.

Headaches can be an excellent example of what happens when the body isn't able to overcome the difficulties that are thrown at it: sitting in the wrong chair at work, having an awkward monitor height, etc. Within the last one or two years, we've had an increasing number of patients arriving with chronic headaches—sometimes acute headaches. These patients have seen many different specialists, neurologists, general practitioners, and physical therapists. Some patients have even considered BOTOX® injections to the suboccipital base of their skull area to help relax some of those muscles. We try to look for more natural solutions to these types of problems.

Headaches respond very well to chiropractic care. We have noticed recently that, due to current technology that people use daily (e.g., cell phones, laptops, tablets, computers at work) and your posture while you're using these devices, a lot of tension develops across the shoulders and in the neck. When these muscles get very tight and tense, that tension can create chronic headaches. The muscle range includes big muscles, such as the upper trapezius, to the little ones, like the suboccipitals and the masseter muscles in the skull/jaw area. The gentle approach of chiropractic treatment can dissolve a lot of this pressure.

The good news is that we see amazing results within four to six weeks, when we employ chiropractic manipulations of the cervical spine and skull. While this method might not work for everybody, the vast majority of patients that we've seen in the last year have responded very well. Sometimes, simple cervical spine manipulation, which most chiropractors employ by hand, can thoroughly address the tension without the need for more aggressive techniques.

We also use some other techniques (when needed) that can be very beneficial, such as active release technique: the soft tissue technique that many of our doctors use in conjunction with manipulation. Finally, we use some ear adjustments that are not used extensively elsewhere. These can help relieve some sinus pressure, and our patients swear by this particular treatment. They sing our praises to their colleagues and friends and are excited to tell their stories. "Hey, I've been dealing with these headaches for more than 20 years, and in just a month and a half, I'm headache-free!"

Many patients are unaware that chiropractic methods can even help with headaches until their friends or co-workers recommend us. Ours isn't a temporary fix. These patients are doing well for the long-term. If you suffer from headaches, make an appointment with a local chiropractor. You may be astonished at the improvement in your quality of life after just a short trial of therapy.

It's important to know that chiropractic care doesn't stop at the spine. When chiropractors manipulate the patient's joints during an adjustment, we reset those joints so they work more efficiently. This manipulation can be on any one of your many joints. Typically, the complaints disappear pretty quickly. Patients appreciate it when they can see their complaints subside over time as the treatment plan is implemented. Patients are pleased when they can see change in the right direction, and that helps them to feel better physically and emotionally.

INTEGRATING WITH OTHER PROFESSIONS

In the past, chiropractic care and traditional medical care were on opposite ends of the healthcare spectrum. We have worked at bringing these two professions together and offering our patients a more patient-centered approach. Our goal has always been to offer our patients the best possible chance for a full recovery, using whatever is best and necessary for our patients. If a massage therapist or physical therapist can accomplish recovery faster than our practice, we refer the patient to the appropriate professional. If the issue appears to be related to blood pressure, we refer the patient to a general practitioner or internist. Patients appreciate that they are at the center of our focus, that we're not just trying to fit their problem into our solution.

In November of 2014, we launched our newest office, using what we call the MD/DC model, which is totally patient-centered. In our newest office, we partnered with a medical doctor, an interventional pain management specialist, a physical therapist, and orthopedic surgeons. There are two types of orthopedic surgery specialists on site. There's a spine specialist and an orthopedic doctor who deals with extremities: knees, shoulders, feet, and elbows. With that model and range of talent, we are prepared to address the patient's needs in almost every way.

This model allows us to guide patients using a better method. The chiropractor can often be the quarterback in the treatment. He designs and calls the plays throughout the care. We're very excited about the new model that we've just started, because it seems to be flourishing—patients come back, and they're excited because they are getting meaningful results. When a patient arrives, we can direct them towards appropriate care in-house and avoid having to refer them across town, possibly delaying necessary treatment. In my estimation, this is the future of chiropractic. I believe that, as we move forward, the patient-centered model and the education model, which help people understand their root issue or issues, will become more common. Within the last five to ten years, the need to understand the underlying issues is the biggest concern that our patients have. By addressing their concerns, we believe we are providing better care to our patients.

Of course, our patients share positive results with their colleagues, their families, and the community as a whole. This system of care is beginning to separate us from some of the former basic models. Our biggest premise is that patients have come to a point where they want to be educated; they want to be partners in their own health care.

Our new model has allowed us to expand within the community, giving us the opportunity to engage patients we might never have seen before. When doctors are working collaboratively, we find it to be very beneficial, and rewarding. So it's a win-win for the patient as well as for the doctors involved. Overall, it's been very positive experience for all of us.

TRAUMA AND INJURY

Personal injury cases show this new model to be especially efficient. People who are involved in motor vehicle accidents or in a slip-and-fall event are often left scratching their heads because they're not sure where to go. Many medical care providers choose to avoid auto accident patients, because they are sometimes limited in how they can help these patients. Contrary to the medical-only model, our specialty (Chiropractic) includes guiding patients through the injury, stabilizing joints, increasing healing time, and helping them to navigate the insurance maze. The insurance is a little bit tricky, but when you've done it for as many years as we have, you learn how to manage it. Not only are we adept at guiding patients through the care they need, but once they're healthy, we can also spare them the after-the-fact headaches of dealing with insurance matters.

Whether it's their own auto insurance or an at-fault insurance, we can guide and direct patients to the right providers sooner rather than later. Again, like a quarterback, the chiropractor is calling the plays. We lead them through the whole process so that their care is better and done without wasting time. Providing care in a timely fashion can be critical. Often, when patients get injured in motor vehicle accidents, they do not get seen and treated quickly—in which case, scar tissue may develop and create more long-term problems.

We strive to quickly address those patients' problems and do the proper diagnostic testing, including any necessary X-rays and MRIs. These tests are all available at our fingertips, so we're generally able to get diagnostic assessments down on a "right here, right now" basis. We stress the importance of diagnostic tests to our patients because accuracy is critical. We also stress the importance of our diagnostic phase to everyone working at the office—every doctor and all of the staff members. "Let's get the diagnoses correct the first time so that we do not have to spin our wheels or turn in circles while we're trying to accurately diagnose the problem."

At the end of the day, we'd rather take the extra time in the beginning to get the diagnoses correct, as opposed to missing crucial pieces and sending the patient in the wrong direction. We want to focus on guiding the patient through the process, whether it's under our care or physical therapy or even with the help of a different kind of specialist. Our goal is to get our patients the help that they need in a timely fashion.

OBJECTIFYING THE SUBJECTIVE COMPLAINT

We are fortunate to have some cutting-edge technology which is able to objectify the subjective complaint. In other words, we want to give our patients some quantifiable illustrations of where we need to go. In terms of technology, we have two touch-friendly systems (MyoVision® and JTECH) to help our patients to see both the current state of their bodies and the goal that they need to reach in order to be healthy.

MyoVision® takes a surface scan in order to show the patient what their muscles are doing. Then, the JTECH system gives us data on range of motion, grip strength, and general muscle health. Combined with the American Medical Association guidelines for normality, we can show to the patients their current state of overall mobility. After ten treatments or so, we can then do a pre-treatment/post-treatment comparison. In this way the patient is empowered by actually seeing his progress. It's not just, "I feel better." The patient can see that he/she "IS" verifiably better.

X-RAYS

We often get questions about our use of x-rays. Even with our wonderful new technology, we still depend heavily upon the old reliable X-ray to help us diagnose and evaluate patient problems. It also helps us to educate our patient about the conditions inside the body. "A picture is worth a thousand words," and so it is with x-ray film, though that still isn't enough. We also have x-ray technicians and radiologists who act as additional sets of eyes to help us identify the root problem, since we are not interested in just treating symptoms. Our goal is to identify the root problem and treat it thoroughly. X-rays help us to do this work.

TECHNOLOGICALLY YOURS

While technology can be used to make chiropractors' jobs easier, it also sends us far too many young patients these days. Younger patients are arriving more and more often with a condition that we call "Text Neck," in which pain is related to the head leaning too far forward over our shoulders (anterior head posture). Text Neck occurs when teenagers or adults spend too much time texting, or working on a laptop at school or the office, with their heads and necks in this particular misalignment. Poor posture mixed with using techno-toys creates too much pressure and eventually causes pain.

Text Neck and carpal tunnel syndrome are both caused by pinched nerves. Without attention to posture while they use technological devices, people may start to feel numbness and tingling in their hands and fingers, or begin to have some grip strength abnormalities. Whether they realize it or not, the sensation in their hands may become altered because of the pressure created as a result of the neck's placement. The medical devices (dynamometer) we use in the office help us identify the pressure moving down the arms from the neck that leads to carpal tunnel syndrome. Sometimes, we can spot it before it becomes symptomatic.

Chiropractic care is perfectly suited to taking the pressure off of those nerves and getting everything working properly again. Using J-Tech scanning and a very conservative treatment plan, we can see the muscular mobility and grip-strength in before-and-after scans, which demonstrate the effectiveness of our treatment.

SCIATICA, PREGNANCY, AND INFANT CARE

Sciatic pain can feel like a lightning bolt was sent down your leg by way of the big muscles of your backside. Sciatica can also take the shape of numbness, tingling, or burning. Whatever shape it takes, it is the result of pressure on a nerve. Unlike other disciplines, we try to avoid things like shots and/or surgery to treat this painful problem. Generally, we can relieve the pressure and the pain if the problem is caught in time.

Another common problem is the low back pain experienced by pregnant women. The extra weight of the baby on the front of the body will cause the mother's back to sway; sciatic pain is very common. We frequently work with the OB-GYN physicians who send us their patients who are affected by sciatic pain. Our conservative approach is optimal here since these mothers cannot take medication for the pain. Many of our pregnant patients report that their deliveries go ex-ceedingly well after they have had chiropractic care along with their obstetric care.

Some may be surprised to learn that when the babies come along, many mothers use chiropractic care to help with ear infections. They do this with the blessings of their pediatricians, because we co-treat with them. Also, if an ear infection can be treated with alternative means using something other than an antibiotic, the long-term benefits are very good for baby and comforting for the mother. The process of birth is a difficult business. Occasionally, the cranial nerves are compressed or otherwise pinched, so the ear infection can be quickly resolved by taking the pressure off of the cranial nerves. Naturally, our approach with infants is extra gentle. As a matter of fact, one might not even see the adjustment being accomplished. The babies love it. Since the gentle touch of our healing hands can bring results very quickly in tiny bodies, babies often respond much faster than adults.

HEARING LOSS

One usually doesn't think about consulting a chiropractor in cases of hearing loss. Nevertheless, you might be surprised to know that one of my most rewarding cases involved helping to restore the hearing of a six-month-old patient. This particular case did not focus on hearing in the initial phases, but it eventually became part of the astonishing overall success of the treatment.

The baby's parents came to my office to discuss their baby's skull, which was set at an odd angle to the spine. They hoped that our gentle adjustments might bring the head into a more usual posture. They had already tried physical therapy to reset the skull—to no avail. So they wanted to consider chiropractic care. In the course of that first interview, they also told me that the audiologist had confirmed that the baby was 100 percent deaf. If a fighter jet landed behind him, he wouldn't know or turn around, because he couldn't hear in either ear. They planned surgery at a later date to see if the procedure might correct the inner ear problems and restore hearing.

I outlined the treatment process that we would use for the parents. I even told them that it was possible that the adjustments might improve the baby's hearing as well as resetting the skull's position on the cervical spine. They seemed dumbfounded and looked at me as if I were a little nuts, but they agreed to the treatments for him anyway.

We started a six- to eight-week treatment program with our extremely gentle adjustment techniques to see if the alignment could be addressed. After about six weeks, we could see that his posture was perfect. He also had 100 percent hearing in his right ear! The right ear and its nerves were under pressure which, once alleviated, made hearing possible. Sadly, the left ear did not respond. The nerve in charge of the left ear was simply stretched too thin to do its job.

The audiologist was astonished, but the initial goal (to re-set the baby's skull) did the trick. Eventually, the parents would have surgery done on the child's left ear, but the right one was fine. This particular case stands out to me as one of the most rewarding experiences that I've had with my career to date.

TREATMENT PLANS

Depending upon the situation and the correction we're aiming to provide, treatment plans can be short-term or more extensive, based on patient needs. Chiropractic care goes far beyond treatment plans, though there is a beginning and end to each plan. Just as dentistry goes beyond filling a tooth or removing those braces, chiropractic care is not just centered on solving the immediate problem. It also includes helping our patients to stay well. In terms of orthodontics, they recommend that you wear your retainer as advised by your doctor to keep the corrections in place. Likewise, in chiropractic care, we want to see our patients from time to time in order to practice maintenance, wellness, and prevention.

Here's another great way to look at treatment plans—changing the oil in your vehicle doesn't excuse you from future maintenance. We recommend body maintenance as well. I often say, "You have one spine. You can either maintain it or let it go." In the long run, it's far more cost-effective to be proactive.

When we ask our patients which of their body's organs is the most important, nine times out of ten, the patient will answer, "The heart." That's not true. Your brain directs the function and the timing of every organ, every muscle, and every cell in your body. This communication primarily happens through the spinal cord. In order for you to remain healthy and operational, you must have a spinal cord that is free to communicate clearly. So, you see, a chiropractor is your body's best friend.

OUR PURPOSE - PREVENTION

In the world of chiropractors, prevention is the ultimate goal. Western medicine is very driven by symptoms. Our branch of the health profession seems to be the only branch in the Western world that bucks the system, so to speak. In a philosophical sense, a patient's medical care depends almost entirely upon the set of symptoms he or she brings to the clinic with them on any given day. In European countries—where socialized medicine makes preventive care essential to reduce long-term costs—they want to keep you healthy in the first place. Prevention has long been the model followed by chiropractic professionals. Our goals do include treating our patients' symptoms, of course, but we also want to keep you well after we've addressed the problem.

There are many ways of ensuring that your health stays at its peak: eat right, exercise regularly, stay hydrated, and get enough sleep. We also think that a monthly massage is important to keep you on track. Unfortunately, many of our patients don't think they have the time for wellness. Busy, successful people are always in a hurry to go somewhere and do something important. They wait to seek treatment until they are in pain. However, ideas and habits are changing in interesting ways.

It is heartening to note that, even in the corporate world, the preventive model is trending upward. Big businesses are beginning to understand that health care can be one of the biggest drains on their profitability as companies. In the interest of preventing health issues, big companies are now employing ergonomic answers, whether it's a desk that can be raised up (making it possible for employees to work while standing at their work stations) or other equipment designed to keep people healthier. Employers are now buying ergonomic chairs and using more ergonomic keyboards and mice. New tools are showing up in the work environment, helping to support the spine and the posture of employees.

As a child, your mother probably told you to stand up straight. That wasn't just because standing up straight makes you look better. Posture is terribly important to your overall health. In an average workday, a person sits in front of a computer for six to eight hours. That's very taxing, not only across your shoulders, but also down your neck. The posture that you use with the monitor and the way your back conforms to the chair can cause your hamstrings to be tight.

Tight muscles and supporting tissue can make exercise more difficult. Ultimately, overlying tight muscles and tissues can make you suffer in other ways, such as thinning bones or even actual bone loss. When our posture is poor, out health tends to follow suit. As chiropractors, we want to encourage better posture and employ techniques for a proactive approach to health care. Our focus is on *health care* so that we can avoid *disease care* in the future.

I believe that we are beginning to see a paradigm shift in our understanding of health care. As health insurance costs go up, many busy people are saying to themselves, "Maybe if I prevent (insert the name of your most intrusive, aggravating condition here) in the first place, I'll be better off in the long run." Well, of course you will. In the next ten to fifteen years we're bound to see a new health-care model in this country and it will center on prevention and wellness. Chiropractic care will probably be a part of that. Perhaps 10 percent of the population uses chiropractic care right now, but I believe that those numbers will reach higher in upcoming years—maybe even up to 80 percent—as people get more proactive and avoid surgeries as a fix-it solution.

WE LOVE MONDAYS

It seems as if everybody hates Mondays, but not at our office. I can't speak for all chiropractors, but our staff may be part of the five percent of the population that doesn't dread Sunday evening. Our profession is so full of surprise and opportunity that every Monday feels like a new adventure. I've been doing this work for ten years, and it feels like I just started. Healing people has to be the most rewarding thing that anybody could do with his time. Our patients appreciate that attitude and it helps with their healing.

It is also very fulfilling to know that educating our patients makes them feel stronger and better able to make good decisions. Of course, this includes not only their physical problems and ways to deal with those issues, but it also includes giving them treatment options and teaching them the ins and outs of insurance issues. This sense of empowerment is important to our model of health care.

When it comes to Monday morning, we look forward to the opportunities that we have to improve lives individually and throughout the entire community. It's not something we simply talk about; it's something we practice on a daily basis.

(This content should be used for informational purposes only. It does not create a doctor-patient relationship with any reader and should not be construed as medical advice. If you need medical advice, please contact a doctor in your community who can assess the specifics of your situation.)

5

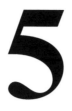

HOLISTIC
CHIROPRACTIC
WELLNESS

by John Gehnrich, D.C.

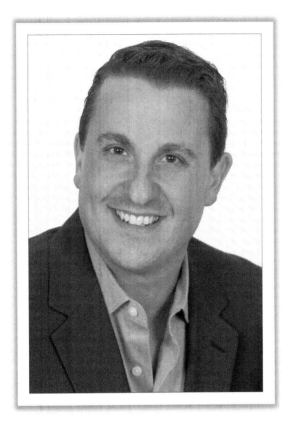

John Gehnrich, D.C.
Rhino Chiropractic & Holistic Wellness Center
Rockville Centre, New York
www.rhinochiropractic.com

John Gehnrich is a passionate Doctor of Chiropractic. He is also a compassionate and intuitive Holistic Wellness Expert, author, lecturer, husband and father. Dr. Gehnrich's own health challenges and miraculous recovery initiated his 20 year journey in the holistic healing arts. Now he is blessed to help others reach their optimal health potential, naturally. Since 2000 Rhino Chiropractic has been serving the community of

Rockville Centre, nestled on the south shore of Long Island, a short train ride from New York City.

Dr. Gehnrich's mission is to offer hope and healing to all he encounters. His unique philosophy is based upon the premise that the body has an innate ability to heal itself. This state of optimal well-being is achieved by first analyzing the underlying cause of your health challenge, and then creating a customized plan of wellness. If you are seeking to get well or to just stay well, Dr. Gehnrich will inspire you to transform your health goals into reality. He in turn is inspired by his beautiful wife Allison and his little angels Alec and Johnny. Dr. John's greatest love is his family, and his greatest passion is to bring healing to his patients and the planet.

HOLISTIC CHIROPRACTIC WELLNESS

AS A CHIROPRACTOR, DO YOU HAVE A UNIQUE VIEW ON WHAT CONSTITUTES GOOD HEALTH?

In my twenty years in the holistic healing arts, I have found that people are taught that health is being pain free and "feeling good." Even though there is a link between how one feels and how healthy they are, in my experience a more accurate indicator is all your bodily systems functioning together in harmony. Oftentimes, a patient will come to me and say, "Doc, it hurts here. It just happened yesterday." In many cases, the root cause of their problem is in a very different location than where their pain is felt. After a thorough history and holistic assessment, we often determine that the underlying cause is an unaddressed physical, chemical, or emotional trauma from the past. Patients are astonished at the intuitiveness and accuracy of a chiropractic assessment. One of the gifts of a good chiropractor is to inspire one's health goals into reality. For those left in hopeless despair, suffering with no cure in sight, rest assured the answer lies within. We as chiropractors can release people's inner power to heal themselves by removing that which interferes with optimal expression of life.

Dorlan's Medical Dictionary tells us that health is a state of wholeness where your body's organs are functioning one hundred percent all of the time. The holistic approach to health does not separate a patient into parts, but rather views the individual as many parts functioning together like the instruments in a symphony. The brain and the spinal cord act as the conductor to every cell, tissue, and organ of the body. Chiropractors help to create the harmony necessary to keep the body functioning as a whole. Though we are empathetic about pain and symptoms, the focus is on removing the interference to allow full expression.

SO, IF I DON'T HAVE ANY PAIN, SHOULD I STILL SEE A CHIROPRACTOR?

In my lectures, I am sure to emphasize that the absence of pain and symptoms does not necessarily indicate good health. In other words, health is not how we feel; it is how we are functioning. Taking a medication to mask something we feel is much like putting tape over a check oil light. Though the immediate signal is blocked, the impending disaster cannot be avoided if the cause is not corrected. By the time many patients seek help, the engine is already on fire. Unfortunately, the first sign of heart disease can be a massive heart attack. The lucky ones will have symptoms: shortness of breath, chest pain, or pain radiating down the arm. The other fifty percent will never have the opportunity to prevent the fatal effects of this disease. Eighty percent of the primary phases of cancer are painless until it's too late. A pea-sized tumor in breast tissue takes up to seven years to develop. You can go to a regular dental checkup and find a cavity that didn't cause any pain. In the same way these health issues can go undetected, spinal alignment and the negative effects of misaligned bones can often escape detection because of their pain-free nature.

In my practice, I evaluate the function of your entire nervous system and the alignment of the vertebral column to determine the state of your health. Through the use of advanced thermographic computer imaging and structural spinal x-rays, we are able to analyze any interference of nerve flow you may not have detected. Health is an accumulation of all of our past lifestyle choices, injuries and traumas, and years of emotional and mental stress. Signals of many of these stressors dissipate as our body accommodates to the repetitive strain of life. Though you may have forgotten the pain of past events, your body stores the memories. As a result, spinal bones misalign (this is called a vertebral subluxation), diminishing the nerve impulses coming from the brain and traveling through the spinal cord, out the spinal bones and through the millions of miles of nerves, to every cell, tissue, and organ in the body. These subluxations often occur painlessly with only ten percent of the spinal nerves sensing pain. The other ninety percent control all of the functions of the body. Subluxations often go without detection due to the asymptomatic nature of spinal misalignments.

Contrary to the popular belief that early detection is the best form of prevention, I would challenge one to think that a proactive approach to a healthy lifestyle is the most empowering action one can take to longevity and quality of life. The lucky ones receive a second chance to take steps toward better health before a condition progresses too far. You may have heard, "If it's not broke, don't fix it." This old way of thinking has led to many of our loved ones exiting this planet prematurely and with great suffering. If we can adopt the idea that "an ounce of prevention is worth a pound of cure," then we can achieve our optimal physical, chemical, and emotional well-being.

A century ago, people simply had teeth pulled when they decayed. The idea of *preventative* dental hygiene did not exist. Now, we go for regular cleanings and checkups. Just as you would visit a dentist to prevent cavities from developing, we want you to maintain your "spinal hygiene" by getting your spine checked for subluxations that may be developing without your knowledge. You can always get dentures and live a perfectly normal and healthy life, but if you allow your spine—which houses your lifeline—to decay, the effects can be irreversible and your spine cannot be replaced.

In chiropractic care, we look at the whole body and help you to resolve the initial crisis so you can "graduate" to pre-ventative wellness visits. We want you to maintain optimal health so that you don't have to come here and say, "Doc, it hurts here." When all of your parts are working together, functioning at optimal potential, then you are truly well.

WE'RE HEARING THE TERM "WELLNESS" A LOT THESE DAYS. AS ONE OF THE LEADING HOLISTIC WELLNESS EXPERTS IN THE FIELD, HOW DO YOU DEFINE WELLNESS?

Wellness is a lifestyle choice. Being truly well is taking an active approach to your health prior to losing it. Wellness is an expression of balance. Chiropractic helps people achieve their optimal physical, chemical and emotional balance by addressing what I like to call the five facets of health: exercise, nutrition, adequate rest, a positive mental attitude, and a properly functioning nervous system.

Most people try to address the first four, but often overlook the fifth and most important. A properly functioning nervous system is the primary goal of chiropractic because there is a direct connection between the nervous system and the function of all the bodily systems. Gray's Anatomy 29th Edition page 4 says, "the nervous system controls and coordinates all organs and structures of the human body."

True wellness is allowing your body to work at its optimal potential by removing interference, making proper lifestyle choices for disease prevention, and working regularly with an open minded, compassionate, and well informed health professional.

By the way, as a chiropractor, I want to re-emphasize that a crucial component of wellness is a well-aligned spine with a properly functioning nervous system free of subluxations.

YOU'VE BEEN USING THE TERM "SUBLUXATION." WHAT ARE THE MAJOR CAUSES AND HOW DOES THIS AFFECT YOUR HEALTH?

The three main causes of subluxation are physical, chemical, and emotional stressors. These stressors cause dis-ease or disharmony in the body, which interferes with your optimal expression of health. Ultimately these subluxations, left unaddressed, will surely take a body in dis-ease to a more permanent state of disease. As a chiropractor, my intention is to seek out and address the underlying cause in each individual case.

When a physical stressor appears to be the cause of the problem, we address it by correcting the underlying structural imbalance in our patients' spines. Many of us have been through traumas over the years including motor vehicle accidents, falls, sports related injuries, and poor postural positioning. Some of the common conditions caused by physical stress are low back pain, neck pain, headaches, disc herniations, sciatica, carpal tunnel syndrome, plantar fasciitis, TMJ, pain between the shoulder blades and radiating down the arm and into the fingers.

Through postural analysis, bilateral gravity assessment, computerized thermal imaging, and full spine structural x-rays, we are able to detect the spinal misalignments (subluxations). This all may sound very "high tech," but we are also very "high touch." We use many hands-on techniques to locate, analyze, and correct vertebral subluxations. Chiropractic adjustments correct subluxations, restore ideal spinal alignment, and actually allow the body to heal itself.

Chemical stresses accumulate in the body either through a build up of toxicity or a deficiency in certain minerals and nutrients. Environmental toxins, processed foods, and harmful medications can be the cause of many misdiagnosed and unresolved health issues. Some of the common conditions caused by neurotoxicity are autoimmune diseases (lupus, RA, MS), mental conditions (ADHD, dementia, Alzheimer's), hormonal disruption (thyroid problems, adrenal fatigue, infertility) and cancers.

Using only the most effective detoxification and cleansing protocols, we stimulate the elimination pathways. Once the body is cleansed, then—and only then—can we begin to introduce the correct balance of nutrition and supplementation. So much emphasis is placed on practicing good nutrition that the importance of clearing the body of harmful toxins is often overlooked. Yes, we are what we eat—but more importantly, we are what we don't eliminate. In fact, no matter how many toxins you eliminate, no matter how clean your diet is, no matter how potent your supplements are, the body must have the correct spinal alignment in order for these things to be truly effective. The adjustment frees communication between the spinal cord and the body's organ systems, allowing them to function at their optimal potential.

The causes of emotional stress are too numerous to list, but what I find in my practice to be the top five are relation-ships, finances, work stress, health issues, and... did I mention relationships?

Whatever the cause, emotional stress creates a neurotoxic effect on the body. The resulting subluxation blocks nerve impulses traveling from the brain and spinal cord out to every cell, tissue, and organ in the body. This disconnection can interfere with the healthy hormones that allow for relaxation and happiness. It can also weaken the immune system, create inflammation, and cause muscle spasms that pull bones out of position. This vicious cycle has to be broken in order to restore emotional balance back to the body. Many patients suffering with anxiety and depression have told me after only a few adjustments that they can feel themselves for the first time in years.

It all starts with awareness. Coming into our office and receiving an adjustment allows patients to reconnect with their own internal place of peace and harmony. I encourage my patients to explore the situations that are causing them stress. Active listening, compassion, and intuition are important in my practice. When my patients open up to me and to their own inner knowing, I can help them to create a stronger internal environment in the midst of tremendous external chaos. This empowers patients so they are no longer seeking a perfect outside world in order to find inner peace. Breathing, meditation, prayer, yoga: all these techniques help people better manage stress, and they also create awareness. I love the expression, "If you give a man a fish, he eats for the day. If you teach a man to fish, he eats for the rest of his life." With every adjustment I clear the interference, so that you can express your body's own healing power.

SO THERE IS A LINK BETWEEN THE SPINAL CORD AND ORGANS. CAN YOU EXPLAIN HOW THAT WORKS?

I refer to this as the neuro-organic connection. The brain and the spinal cord are the master control center of the body, but the nervous system is only complete when nerves that exit the spine connect to the organs without interference. Remember, Gray's Anatomy teaches that every cell, tissue, and organ in the body is connected to the brain through the nerves. A misalignment of the spinal vertebrae and discs, called subluxation, may cause a disconnection within the nervous system which then affects the organs and their functions. The basic premise of chiropractic is that these subluxations cause dis-ease in the body, which ultimately may lead to disease. It is essential that your spine be checked regularly by your chiropractor for subluxations and adjusted into the correct alignment in order to remove the interference and free every part of your body, your *whole* body, to function properly. This is why people say, what, does chiropractic cure everything? I say, it allows your body to express itself at its optimal potential so that you can be healthy.

When people come in seeking only an answer to a particular health problem, often we find a hidden connection that is revealed when the subluxation is freed. The neck region can relate to migraine headaches, sinus and allergies, TMJ, and thyroid conditions. The mid-back area connects to the heart, lungs, and stomach, which can be related to one's blood pressure, asthma, and heartburn. Finally, the low back. Besides low back pain and sciatica, misalignment of this segment of the spine can lead to constipation, colitis, PMS, and infertility.

There was actually a patient who came to me a few months ago suffering with horrible migraine headaches, disc herniations in her neck and low back, and sciatica. She came in only seeking to rid herself of the debilitating pain. She said, "I tried everything and nothing has worked. Please fix me." I told her that unlike traditional approaches, chiropractic does not aim to cure, treat, or fix. You cure bacon, you treat carpets, and you fix flats, but I as a chiropractor help release the subtle substance of your soul so you may reach your innate healing potential.

After examining her spine and detecting numerous subluxations, the organic connection revealed itself. She saw that each of her issues--sinus and allergies, asthma, heartburn, constipation, and painful menstrual cycles—seemed related to a subluxation at a specific level of the spine. When we reviewed the structural abnormalities on her x-rays, the correlation became solidified in her mind. She even said, "A picture speaks a thousand words. You can't argue with that." Then we created a specific care plan, starting her on the first step of the journey thousands have taken before her. Now, even though her pain is gone, what she is most excited about is that she is no longer dependent on drugs to help her face the day. She wakes each morning with renewed hope, a new sense of freedom, and a newfound confidence in her own healing potential.

I'm seeing more and more patients starting to recognize their potential for healing. They come in open to a new way of thinking because of their frustration with the old methods. For years, a majority of people who entered our practice had come in with musculoskeletal complaints (neck pain, back pain, headaches, sciatica and disc herniations). Now, more patients come to us seeking a holistic approach. This new way of thinking about their health empowers them to take an active role in the healing process through lifestyle changes and corrective chiropractic adjustments.

WHY DO YOU THINK THE CONCEPTS OF "THE ORGANIC CONNECTION" AND HOLISTIC CHIROPRACTIC HAVE NOT REACHED THE MAINSTREAM YET?

Honestly, this concept is not new. Hippocrates, the father of modern medicine, stated almost 2500 years ago, "Look well to the spine for the cause of disease." Thomas Edison said, "The doctor of the future will give no medicine, but will interest the patient in the care of the human frame, in diet, and in the cause and prevention of disease."

Acupuncturists have long been healing all types of ailments using needles to free blocked energy channels, and Ayurvedic healers have helped people regain their health using roots, twigs, and herbs. These ancient healing arts have long accessed the body's innate ability to heal itself. What the body needs more than intervention is simply no interference. Then it is able to do what it is intended to. I believe chiropractic has become the most logical, time efficient, and cost effective approach to natural healing this planet has ever known. My mission is to educate every man, woman and child about this life-altering practice, so that they may come to experience the total health and well being that can be achieved through chiropractic.

One of the most glaring problems with our current status quo is that drugs introduced in order to remove a problem (as we all know from those drug commercials with the endless horrifying warnings) tend to create problems of their own. There is no pill, potion, or lotion on the market today that can touch a candle to the power of a chiropractic adjustment.

Chiropractic in the mainstream just makes sense as a drugless solution. It removes the interference which caused the problem your medicine was meant to remove—and whether that drug was successful or not in resolving that issue, it most likely introduced a whole new host of problems to your system; all of which could have been avoided in millions of cases if chiropractic were recommended as often as drugs.

WHAT DO YOU THINK OF THE CURRENT STATE OF HEALTH CARE?

The U.S. ranks low in health compared to the rest of the world. The World Health Organization puts us at 37th of all industrialized nations. Our model of health care is truly "sick care." One typically waits for an illness or disease in order to seek medical assistance. Very rarely do we see patients going to their medical doctor saying "Doc, I feel great. Do you have anything you can give me to keep me healthy?" Of course we all know the answer to that.

Chiropractic does not treat, cure, or fix any problem; rather, through realigning the vertebra and removing the interference in the nervous system, it allows the body the optimal environment to heal itself. Modern medicine has saved millions of lives through emergency medical intervention and life-saving procedures. We believe if one can stay free from subluxations, the need for those interventions would be drastically reduced. Ultimately, the prevention of dis-ease is far superior to the treatment of the end-stage disease.

While many in the medical community have not embraced this new paradigm, some progressive doctors are getting on board. They are starting to refer patients that haven't seen resolution of their health challenges through the traditional Western methods. They love the fact that their patients report improvement of a long-standing health complaint for the first time in years after only a few adjustments.

These cutting-edge physicians know that many medical practices, such as injections, surgeries, and the prescribing of drugs, are performed from the outside in, administered to the body—whereas holistic chiropractic directs a specific adjustment to the spine which allows the body to heal itself from the inside out. I always ask my patients, "Can you tell me who the greatest doctor in the world is?" I tell them, "I am" which always gets a laugh. Then I say, "And you are the best doctor in the world, for you." We were born with the innate ability to heal. My job is to release the maximum flow of innate potential so you are able to reconnect with the doctor within.

SO FAR, YOU'VE SHARED A LOT ABOUT CHIROPRACTIC BEING ABOUT CLEARING INTERFERENCE, BUT WHAT ABOUT PEOPLE WHO JUST SUFFER FROM COMMON PAINS AND SPINAL PROBLEMS?

Lower back and sciatic pain, neck pain and pain radiating down the arm into the fingers, migraine headaches and TMJ, disc bulging and herniations: these are as common to my profession as cavities are to dentistry. Like a dentist checking for cavities that lead to tooth decay, my job as a chiropractor is to locate and correct the subluxations that create many of the unwanted health conditions that bring you to my office. These common ailments that are likely to affect you at one time or another, and seem to plague a majority of your friends and neighbors, can be avoided by receiving a simple, specific and painless evaluation by a chiropractor trained in the science and art of detecting and correcting subluxations.

When folks come in with pain, we work together to stop the pain—but really, we are working to clear the interference that is causing the pain and a variety of other symptoms as well. People who have come in for pain more recently have been aware that there is so much more there than just a bulging disc or a headache, and they are looking for so much more than a quick fix. I always said, "If patients knew what I knew they would do what I do." The exciting thing is, they are starting to find out. They are starting to understand.

No matter how we are feeling, my family and I get checked for subluxations once a week to maintain a healthy spine and prevent many of the unnecessary health conditions plaguing our society. It will be interesting to continue to watch the difference chiropractic care has made in the health of my children. My wife and I have had numerous health challenges through the years, from lower back and neck pain and torn rotator cuffs to colitis, allergies, and PMS—by the way that last one was my wife's! My children, on the other hand, have been adjusted since they were born to prevent any potential future issue. Thank God (and chiropractic), they have experienced few of the health challenges we see in children of their age group at my office. I've been fortunate enough to raise children who are free of the effects of ear infection, asthma, colic, and ADD.

HOW IMPORTANT IS GOOD POSTURE TO YOUR OVERALL HEALTH?

One of the most common spinal issues we work to resolve is, quite simply, poor posture. Posture is the window to the spine and affects and reflects your health. In the 1920s, Henry Winsor performed autopsies that proved the irrefutable correlation between diseased organs and the spinal column. He found that the greater the misalignment or curvature of the spine, the more severe the disease in the corresponding part of the body.

Scientists continue to research and validate the organic connection that Dr. Winsor proved. For years, his work was largely unknown as so much was at stake for the drug companies and the rest of mainstream medicine. Because of this, many doctors remain unaware of this crucial connection.

Over the years, the link has been proven again and again. Alfred Breig, a neurosurgeon, was widely celebrated for his work linking spinal health with overall health. He actually won the Nobel Prize for revealing the importance of a healthy spinal curve to a healthy body and the unfortunate opposite that occurs with a reversing spinal neck curve. People who have a reduction or reversal in the ideal C-shaped curve of the neck have higher levels of disease in their bodies. A reduction in compression, stretching, or cord tension on your spinal cord will vastly improve your health.

In 1994, a research article in the *American Journal of Pain* indicated that posture affects and moderates every physiological function from breathing to hormone production. Poor posture can lead to conditions as varied as spinal pain, headaches, mood disorders, and asthma. Pulse and lung capacity are normal functions that can be affected by posture. People may think it is "normal" for a senior citizen to develop arthritis or a stooped posture, but such abnormalities in spinal health can cause dangerous conditions like high blood pressure or reduced lung capacity. Though they are common, there are no "normal" spinal abnormalities. Often, they are caused by years of neglect and if addressed early enough, can be corrected with chiropractic adjustments.

DO YOU SEE A LOT OF CHILDREN WITH SCOLIOSIS?

Oh, yes, and many of them have already developed asthma, allergies, and ear infections. It is best to start improving posture in childhood. It is not just safe for children to have adjustments from the time they are born; it is crucial to their lifelong spinal health. Often, children will be brought to me when they have already been gravely affected by the effects of poor spinal health. Many of them may be at a point where they have had recommendations of spinal rod surgery to straighten the back. This procedure is a last resort due to its invasiveness, whereas regular chiropractic visits will slowly and gently reintroduce the proper alignment.

These specific spinal adjustments retrain the ligaments and nerves to find their correct position, which allows for reduction of symptoms and better nerve flow. We bring the spine back into proper alignment—and we are not just guessing. We analyze the posture, with a Spinal Analysis Machine, check for weight imbalances on a Bilateral Gravity Assessment scales and measure the area and severity of pinching nerves (subluxation) using a Tytron Spinal Thermography Imaging device.

HOW DO CHILDREN GET THESE MISALIGNMENTS AT SUCH A YOUNG AGE, AND HOW DO YOU HELP?

Structural corrective chiropractic can help a child who comes to us with scoliosis, but children who receive adjustments from birth will see the benefits from the first time a chiropractor helps them through an incredible traumatic process—birth. So much pressure has been placed on that baby's neck that visible trauma is evident on the first two neck bones. Of course, we do not add to that pressure—there is no need to fear that we will be twisting or maneuvering an infant or child's spine. Children respond to a very light touch, so we do not use much force at all.

By the way, when I perform an adjustment, in no way am I displacing or causing degenerative change to your bones. Repeated adjustments will cause no harm whatsoever, to adults or children. On the contrary, it slows the degenerative changes of arthritis. It may be reassuring to people who are nervous about injury that we chiropractors pay less than one percent of what medical doctors pay in insurance for the same level of coverage! That is how safe it is. Our adjustments are not like the manipulating and snapping that occur when you crack your knuckles or have someone untrained crack your back, often resulting in harmful hypermobility of the joint. We are in fact adjusting, with a purpose. With our hands or other tools, we realign a specific misalignment that we detected through thorough investigation of your spine.

With children, we use a lighter force that is often soundless. For adults who are uncomfortable with the "cracking" sound, we can use a lighter touch or instruments to achieve the same result. However, have no fear—the sound that you hear is only the escape of gas built up in the joint, similar to the sound you hear when you crack your knuckles.

When children come to us from day one, they often become lifelong patients who are healthy and largely free of structural problems. When a child comes to us later with scoliosis, or a related organic issue like asthma, colitis, or thyroid dysfunction, we work to restore that ideal healthy spine through structural corrective chiropractic. I always say to the parents, "Don't leave your children home to develop the same problems you have."

SO IF YOU VISIT A CHIROPRACTOR, DO YOU HAVE TO THEN GO FOR THE REST OF YOUR LIFE?

Just as you take care of the alignment of your teeth, or your car's alignment, you should be sure to tend to the alignment of your spine. Your spine, brain, and spinal cord make up the "life line" that controls every cell and organ in your body.

You brush your teeth twice a day and visit the dentist once or twice a year, right? It only makes sense that you should regularly visit a chiropractor to take care of your spine. If you are not in any pain, and if you never visit an office like mine, you will likely not realize that you have spinal misalignment that could potentially cause sciatic nerve pain, numbness and tingling in your hand, or misaligned spinal discs. Unfortunately, you may not realize that you should have your spine checked on a regular basis just like you go for your dental checkups, routine medical exams, and blood work.

When a patient asks about coming to see me "for the rest of his life" I ask him, "When do you plan to stop brushing your teeth, eating well, or changing the oil in your car?" "If you start seeing a benefit, then it's a good investment in your health." You come to me because you want to get healthy. Together we create a customizable plan of action. We will make it work for you, and once you feel the benefit, you are going to *want* to come as often as necessary to maintain your health and of course to catch and clear any interference before it's too late.

CAN YOU EXPAND UPON HOW CHIROPRACTIC HELPS YOUR BODY HEAL ITSELF? HOW WILL I FEEL AS YOU TAKE ME THROUGH THE PROCESS OF HEALING?

A major premise of chiropractic is that the body has an innate intelligence that self-regulates, self-heals, and self-corrects. Just as a cut hand bleeds, experiences pain, and then begins to heal by forming a scab, all done without any conscious thought or intention, the whole body has the ability to heal itself once you clear the interference. You don't even have to think about it. The power that made the body heals the body.

Since 1895, the all-encompassing benefits of a chiropractic adjustment have helped millions regain their lives. These spinal bones that have been misaligned for years, often without detection, can wreak havoc on your well-being. A skilled chiropractor will hone in on the specific subluxations that are affecting your health.

Sometimes, people feel worse before they feel better. If the body is toxic and out of balance, some patients feel "retracing", which is the body clearing out old traumas and toxins, like peeling the layers of an onion. If you get food poisoning, the vomiting and diarrhea you experience is not the sickness. It is the cleansing. You are ejecting the poison; this is a healthy response. If your body did not respond in this unpleasant way, you would become even sicker and could even die. A healthy body runs a fever to burn off toxins.

If your body gets a great adjustment and starts clearing out toxins, you may experience some discomfort such as numbness in the fingers, not because the adjustment has caused a problem, but because you are getting oxygen back in the farthest reaches of your body! The feeling is finally returning!

Before my patients get their first adjustment, I always inform before I perform. I explain to them the possible responses they might experience. A majority of our patients (85-90%) will have an amazing experience! Less pain, more energy, improved range of motion, a great night's sleep. Most of the remaining minority of patients will have no change and 1-2% may have what we call a "re-tracing" event. This is when a long forgotten symptom from the past can rear its ugly head. Some patients have come to me saying "this other chiropractor made me worse," but the concept of re-tracing was never explained to them. I tell them that their body is waking up and trying to heal itself of an old unresolved issue. You may need to feel it to heal it, but in these very rare cases we will modify our game plan to slow down the process for this patient and take a more gradual approach to their healing. As with any caring and knowledgeable health practitioner there should be open and honest two-way communication between patient and doctor.

WHAT OTHER CONDITIONS HAS CHIROPRACTIC HELPED WITH?

When the Spanish flu epidemic of 1918 killed millions of people throughout the US and the world, chiropractors were right there on the front lines healing people. Our expertise has proved essential in dealing with a world health crisis, because we go to the root of the disease and clear the body to function at its highest level. Chiropractors can even bring people, by the thousands, back from the very lowest level of functioning.

Then there are the kinds of health problems most people think of when they think of chiropractic, like arthritis. In some cases, an adjustment slows down and prevents the debilitating effects of arthritis. In our office, we work on the areas above and below the bone decay to prevent arthritis from taking hold. We have helped so many people resume the normal activities they have been missing. I love when a patient who has been suffering with arthritis comes in on a Monday and I ask how the weekend was and they say, great! I went bowling or I went skiing or I gave my grandson a piggyback ride. There's no better feeling in the world.

Maintaining joint health and mobility is so important to our active lives. But an adjustment to a joint has some surprising benefits too. Realigning the joints can affect both the joint's mobility and the function of various organ systems because parts of the brain are stimulated by adjustments. Messages sent through the joint into the spinal cord and brain affect neurological function. People with certain types of neurological conditions such as Parkinson's or MS can show some tremendous improvements from spinal adjustments.

People are really surprised by some of the health issues that can be addressed with our help. One of the most amazing examples is the result of the first chiropractic adjustment. It was performed by D.D. Palmer in Davenport, Iowa on a deaf janitor, and it helped him to regain his hearing! He could suddenly hear street noise for the first time in years.

I have helped women struggling with infertility to conceive. Most often they have had undetected subluxations in the lower spine leading to the reproductive area. I have had the great honor of holding a baby, knowing I helped clear the way for her to enter this world.

Parents have seen great miracles, like little Brandon's mom. She brought him into our office when he was having problems with the tubes he'd had in his ears since he was six months old. His mom was crying because she'd been told he would need another surgery. We began to adjust him for subluxations in the top part of his neck, and recommended he reduce the amount of dairy and white flour in his diet. After only eight weeks of adjustments and some chemical clearing, Brandon's mom came to me, thrilled: he did not need the surgery!

I want to reiterate: because chiropractic gets at the root of the dis-ease, because it clears the interference in your body, because it taps into the organic connection, because it brings your whole body back into healthy alignment and allows for optimal flow of all that is good, it can help heal your life. No matter what you are suffering.

SO PLEASE SUM IT UP FOR ME. WHY SHOULD I GO SEE A CHIROPRACTOR?

I often wonder whether we really have a wellness model in health care today. It seems to me that our current model is actually based on sick care. Too often, people will not go to the doctor until there is a problem, and that is too late. There are inroads in proactive wellness: insurance companies are giving discounts to folks who don't smoke, who go to the gym and whose blood levels are within a healthy range, but proactive wellness is not a concept truly embraced by the current system.

The only true health reform is self-reform. You have to make a choice to be proactive about your own health. When is the last time you visited the doctor when you felt good? You go to the chiropractor because you do not want to wait to be sick. You do not want to get to the point of needing drugs or surgery.

All of us doctors swear to uphold the oath, "First, do no harm." You do not want to have to use an intervention that exposes you to all kinds of new risks for a questionable benefit. Our aim in chiropractic is to protect you from the harmful effects of these last-resort procedures. We help you to attain optimal health with virtually no risk.

It sounds amazing but it's true. I love the skeptics. My best patients are the reformed skeptics! Once they get results, they cannot refute the effectiveness of chiropractic and they shout it from the mountaintops. They wonder why their doctors never told them about us. In fact, these days, some of our best reformers are medical doctors, orthopedists, and neurologists who now see the benefit of chiropractic care. We have often had an uneasy relationship with the medical community over the years, especially in the 1960s when we began to take a substantial portion of the market share. The AMA unsuccessfully tried to discredit us, but since the Supreme Court validated the legitimacy of our profession, and since thousands have attested to miracles like those I described, and since doctors themselves have been coming for adjustments and seeing results in the patients they've sent our way, we are proud to stand at the forefront of what I hope is a change in the way we think about health care.

We have certainly seen in our office that structurally correcting a spinal misalignment is a crucial part of establishing your health so that you do not have to resort to sick care. No matter how well you eat or how much you exercise, if you are out of alignment, the pressure on your nervous system will prevent you from being at your true best. The interference caused by subluxations need to be corrected.

WHAT SETS YOU APART? WHAT WILL I GAIN BY SEEING DR. JOHN GEHNRICH AT RHINO CHIROPRACTIC?

I am not a chiropractor who sees you one time, and you leave with no pain, and I say, "OK, see you when you hurt again." Then I would be part of the sick care system. I want to see you regularly. I want to adjust you so you can maintain your optimal health, not just to get rid of the back, neck, and head pain, or pain from auto- or work-related injuries. I subscribe more to the original model of chiropractic. Remember, the first chiropractic adjustment resulted in a deaf man hearing. I am all about the miracle stories, and I even have one of my own.

I am not here to cure you, or even treat any one condition or disease you may have. When I remove your subluxations, I will help to create the right conditions for your entire body to heal itself. By analyzing the structure of your spine and adjusting it, I correct specific misalignments to achieve a structural change at the most basic level. No medical treatment you can find goes this deep.

I will take the journey with you. We will dig deep everywhere, as you are ready. We will clear you out with adjustments as well as nutritional and lifestyle changes. We will get at the emotional root of your health problems. I will bring my best listening, my compassion, and my passion to every session.

WHERE DID YOUR PASSION FOR CHIROPRACTIC COME FROM? AND WHAT DRIVES IT NOW?

I was inspired by a boy. He was born against all odds, to a woman who benefitted from chiropractic. Back when she was in her twenties, and this is way back, over 40 years ago--she was vacationing in Europe and lugging around a big bag. She felt a pop in her lower back. Whatever had happened there caused her menstrual cycle to stop. Back in the US, a medical doctor wanted to put her on birth control pills to regulate her menstrual cycle, but her sister got her in to see a chiropractor, who said, "We should be able to get your cycle regulated within a month."

A few adjustments and some supplements, and her cycle was back! She was so thrilled and so grateful that when she gave birth to a daughter one year later, she named her chiropractor the godfather. This child had no health issues, but four years later a son was born with a tumor the size of a baseball. His intestines were telescoped into each other. He had an obstruction, and when he was six months old they had to resection his colon, saving his life, but the anesthesia and the multiple medications had taken their toll, and the little boy cried for the first two years of his life. Even though he was in the world because a chiropractor had helped his mother, he had never been to one himself.

About four years later, his mother noticed he was breathing through his mouth and sitting really close to the TV. She knew something was off, and brought him to an ENT who found that his Eustachian tubes were closed and his tonsils and adenoids were extremely swollen. Under the guidance of medical doctors, his mom opted to have her son's tonsils and adenoids removed and tubes drilled into his ears—measures too often taken, still to this day.

This boy reacted very poorly to the anesthesia, but he had to go back for more, because the tubes wouldn't take. From the age of four until he was eight, his body kept rejecting the tubes and the doctor would put them back in, one ear then the other then the other again. Finally, when he turned nine, he was given the option of surgery in the office with no anesthesia. He decided he would brave it, and just hold his mother's hand for comfort. They cut open his ear drum and drilled the tube in—and he nearly broke his mother's hand, but all that suffering would be for nothing, because his body rejected the tubes again.

As he got older, this boy developed bronchial asthma and allergies. He was given multiple medications that limited him.

He had to take frequent breaks from his martial arts classes to use his inhaler so that he could continue training.

So, let's fast forward to my practice now. Remember little Brandon? After a few adjustments and some nutritional changes, he did not need tubes anymore. Because of chiropractic, in just eight weeks, he was able to go back to swimming, his favorite activity, in no time.

Then there was Vincent. Another miracle story. Mom was in tears when she brought him to me. He didn't have bronchial asthma, but severe asthma that he was being treated unsuccessfully using Prednisone and an Albuterol inhaler. He sat before me full of steroids and still breathing through his mouth and his mom said, "Can we give this a try?" I adjusted his neck and by the third visit, he was vomiting Albuterol and tons of pink medicine. These specific adjustments realigned his spine, ridding him of toxins and liberating him from the grip of asthma.

This is why I'm so impassioned about chiropractic. It's the Brandons and the Vincents and all the other children made healthy, and all the children made possible, and it all started with one child—me. That was me, on the sidelines in Tae Kwon Do. That was me, sick until the age of 16, having never seen the chiropractor who could have cleared all that inter-ference, all those chemicals. I could have healed myself had someone helped me clear the way. As an adult, I have a choice. It is my lifelong goal to heal myself and others, and to tell people the truth about chiropractors so no one has to suffer unnecessarily like I once did.

I want to go out into the world and relieve all the suffering. I have gone on some incredible mission trips. In Panama I joined other chiropractors to help the people there and I saw miracles you read about in the bible: deaf people hearing, blind people seeing, lame people walking, babies sleeping through the night for the first time in months! I adjusted 7,000 people in one week. It was amazing to have some of these miracles performed through me—not from me, but through me. It was an honor to help during the aftermath of 9/11. I wanted to help the first responders as they came out of the thick of it—to balance them before they went back into that horrible scene so they could stay healthy and physically strong when they had no time to emotionally process any of it. We go into soup kitchens, we helped after Katrina and in Haiti and following other natural disasters around the world. We are chiropractors for humanity, changing the world one spine at a time.

Most of all, I want to help you, the individual. My passion is to help you and your family so, God willing, you can live a healthy and vibrant life filled with abundance and prosperity. What I want, more than anything, is to bring peace, joy, and happiness to the world—and to you, my patient and my partner on this mission.

(This content should be used for informational purposes only. It does not create a doctor-patient relationship with any reader and should not be construed as medical advice. If you need medical advice, please contact a doctor in your community who can assess the specifics of your situation.)

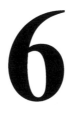

6

CHIROPRACTIC CARE - FROM THE INSIDE OUT

by Ellan Duke, D.C.

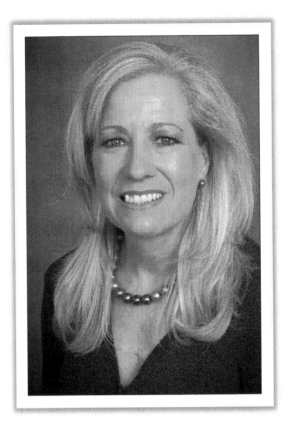

Ellan Duke, D.C.
River Hills Chiropractic & Wellness Center
Jacksonville, Florida
www.riverhillsclinic.com

Dr. Ellan Duke is a Nutritionist, Chiropractor and Certified Sports Physician. She has been the director of River Hills Clinic in Jacksonville Florida for the past 25 years.

Dr. Ellan Duke has been serving her community on the Mayor's Council of Fitness and Well Being for many years. She is on the advisory board for the YMCA and the advisory board for The City Rescue Mission.

Dr. Duke is the facilitator of the Local Christian Chiropractic Association. She is a member of the American and Florida Chiropractic Associations as well as the Easter Seals. She is also a teacher for the American Red Cross.

Dr. Duke develops Nutrition and fitness programs for weight loss, detox, allergies, infertility, hormone balancing, anti-aging, diabetes and cancer. She has been published many times and speaks to groups on a regular basis about healthy living.

She has been married to her husband Thomas for 30 years. Thomas is an Architect who also practices in Jacksonville. They have four grown sons and one darling granddaughter.

CHIROPRACTIC CARE – FROM THE INSIDE OUT

I graduated from high school at age 17 and finished my doctorate degree at age 25. As a young physician, I was a little nervous about performing to perfection. I opened River Hills Chiropractic and Wellness Center in Jacksonville, Florida in 1989. I was so excited to finally pursue my passion. My desire was simply to facilitate healing—in mind, body and spirit—for as many as I could.

I remember my first phone conference with the head of ICU at our nearby Memorial Hospital. I tried extra hard to display noticeable confidence and intelligence in hopes to earn a relationship and respect as a colleague and peer. Every word was significantly thought out as to give the best possible impression. When I had finished my conversation with Dr. Paul, my performance slipped as I briefly took off my doctor hat and put on my mommy hat. At that time I was the mother of two small boys under the age of three. In my final words of closing I said, "Doc, it was a pleasure speaking with you. Night night." We then both hung up our phones and I immediately thought in my head, "Oh My Gosh, did I just say 'night night'?" Did my A+ score in sophistication suddenly descend to a C minus? I was haunted by this blunder for many days.

Comically, as life unfolds, the next year this doctor became not only a patient of mine but a close friend. He left Jacksonville to teach at the University of Miami in multiple organ transplants and later at Emory University. Over the years I have had the pleasure of treating many other physicians, local politicians, and other prominent people in our community. I share this to suggest to chiropractors beginning in their careers to stand tall and confident in the gift we have to share. I have seen so many seemingly miraculous outcomes. No one can put a price tag on better health. Bless and Be Blessed!

I am honored to be included in this special book. It warms my heart to know that the proceeds from this project will be donated to Kiwanis International, a service organization. I've been involved in Kiwanis since I was a girl. My best friend, Sharon Hafner, and I entertained at the 1981 installation of officers program. I was also proud to be selected in 11th grade as the "sweetheart" of our all-male Key Club of Vanguard High School. I went on to be an officer in the co-ed Circle K Club of Palm Beach State College. These are the youth divisions of Kiwanis. In a very real way, the Kiwanis taught me to serve the community and have fun doing it, from painting widows' houses to helping with pancake breakfasts. That was, of course, before gluten became so unpopular. Once again, I am delighted to be contributing to their efforts.

For my part of this collection of chiropractic tidbits, I'd like to give a sort of brief overview of my career path so as to reminisce with old friends and hopefully welcome new ones. I love sharing the ways in which Chiropractic enables me to help others and to enrich my community. I have been the owner and director of River Hills Clinic for the past 25 years. In addition to chiropractic we provide massage, acupuncture, physical therapy, personal training, yoga, Pilates, and other fitness classes. We also offer Nutritional Counseling for weight loss, detox, anti-aging, hormone balance, infertility, cancer, and diabetes. On a personal note, I have been married to my wonderful husband, Thomas Duke, for 30 years. He has his own architectural firm and is currently the president of our local chapter of the AIA. We have four grown sons and one darling granddaughter.

WHAT IS CHIROPRACTIC CARE ALL ABOUT?

Right now is an exciting time to be a chiropractor because it has become so popular. One of the biggest reasons is that folks are living so much longer and we all want those additional years to be of good quality. In order to extend and enrich life, people are trying to get back to natural health-care solutions, like not taking as many prescriptions and avoiding surgical procedures that might be unnecessary. People are also beginning to understand that chiropractic care is one of those proactive and preventive activities that can improve not only musculoskeletal health but also systemic health. In fact, most medical doctors recommend that you get your spine checked just as regularly as you get your teeth cleaned—every six months.

Basically, all chiropractors do the same thing. They palpate and observe the spine to make sure that everything is in the right position. Second, they check that the spine is flexible, not seized up or bound up in any way. In other words, if you bent over to touch your toes, the spaces between all 24 of your vertebrae should open up a little, giving you lots of flexibility. If ten of your vertebrae are doing the work of the other 14, that's a big problem. Displaced or jammed vertebra will wear down in the same way that coarse sand paper can wear away hardwood. Eventually, this kind of erosion can become degenerative arthritis, which causes pain and inflammation. The good news is that most of this damage is avoidable with regular spinal check-ups.

EARLY INFLUENCES

I was steered into this wonderful career by a sequence of events from my childhood. After my father's service in the US Navy, he worked as a mechanical engineer. A financial recession caused him to close his engineering firm and open a convenience store in the little community of Rives Junction, Michigan. We lived in a two bedroom apartment above the store. All six children shared the same room. We'd still label those as the "good ole days."

For some time, our family of eight consumed a lot of items that Dad stocked on those store shelves. This was mostly processed food that was overloaded with artificial flavorings and coloring and preservatives that gave it a five-year shelf life. Since then, scientists' research on processed foods has revealed that those kinds of foods don't just harbor empty calories. Some significant negative impact upon your overall health accompanies poor food choices. We jokingly refer to those empty calories as "Frankenfood".

Looking back, it was not surprising when nearly everyone in our family slowly became fat and sick and tired. Our eating trends began to change when my mother discovered the writings of Adelle Davis, who was a pioneer in the field of nutrition for wellness. As my mom began to apply some of what she read, everybody's health began to improve. Soon after this, we sold the store in Michigan and moved to a farm in Ocala, Florida. Led by my city slicker dad who was raised in Detroit, our family of eight learned to live off the land. We planted gardens, gathered chicken eggs, milked the cows and separated the cream to shake it into butter. Intrigued with using food as medicine I received my pre-med bachelor's degree in Nutritional Counseling and Sciences. I have really enjoyed helping patients find natural solutions to their health conditions. Nutritional counseling has always been a large part of my chiropractic career.

NUTRITION 101

With the assistance of the internet, it is now much easier for patients to research which nutrients help to maintain good health and or help your body to heal certain ailments. However, this research often ends in a lot of effort with little to no results. The first problem is that we now live in a much more toxic environment with depleted soils. Even when we go out of our way to eat healthy and clean, our food sources simply do not contain the quantity of nutrients that they used to. This requires us to supplement our diets. The second problem lies with the fact that so much of what is sold in our country as natural health care remedies is watered down junk that has little to no impact on a person's health. Staying on top of what is actually good for you or even useful is a continuous job.

As the famous nutritionist Lindsey Duncan would say, "We must be strategic about taking care of our health." He is the founder and formulator of the Genesis Pure Company, which provides some of the highest quality products available. In our clinic, we use mostly these and Standard Process whole food supplements. However, supplementation (no matter how high the quality might be) should not replace nutritious whole foods. Over time, the right whole foods will give you the best results because whole foods contain important enzymes that are usually lost in processing. Enzymes tell your body what to do with the food you ingest.

The nutrient value of foods is measured on the ORAC or ANDI scale: the higher the number, the better the food is for you. While grocery shopping, hopefully you will select not necessarily the ones with the least calories but instead the ones with the most actual nutrition. Items with the highest ORAC and ANDI numbers are commonly referred to as "super foods" which are the best at feeding and fueling our body machines. Greens and berries are usually the highest in nutritional density. Goji berries are close to the top; they're nicknamed "The Happy Berry" for their impact on mental clarity and mood enhancement. (Before consenting to a long-term prescription of antidepressants, first try goji berries.) Kale usually wins in the "greens" department, coming in at 1770 on the ORAC scale. Try to eat kale several times each week.

Also, don't forget Mila! Mila is a special blend of chia seeds that measures a whopping 1157 on the ORAC scale and ranks as one of my favorite whole foods. Mila contains all three food categories of fats, carbohydrates, and protein and can also help with weight-loss. In 2011, I helped Dr. Bob Arnot (the Chief Medical Correspondent for NBC and CBS networks at the time) to facilitate a detox/weight loss research project using Mila and other whole foods to make meal-replacement smoothies. Those who participated lost an average of one-half to one pound per day. One gentleman in St. Augustine lost 65 pounds in two months. Our amazing results are published in Doctor Arnot's latest book, called *The Aztec Diet*.

EDUCATION ALWAYS

Along with loving the field of nutrition, I have always had a strong desire to specialize in helping those with physical handicaps. This was largely because of my little brother who was born with Cerebral Palsy and hard of hearing. At a very young age, I was involved with the Easter Seals, first as a volunteer then as a paid counselor at Camp Challenge, which is a summer camp for those with physical and mental disabilities. With this emphasis, I began college classes to major in physical therapy. Around this time, I accepted a position in the chiropractic clinic of Dr. Maria Romanelli. She would become my mentor and lifelong friend. After seeing some amazing results in that clinic, I changed my major to chiropractic and began the additional 8-year journey of schooling, and I have never looked back. To this day, I thank God for guiding me to this occupation which has been so rewarding for three decades.

SOME EXTRAORDINARY PATIENTS

In our clinic, we have taken care of many patients with difficult physical disabilities. While it's true that you can probably never get patients without legs to independently walk again, if you can alleviate even a little of their discomfort, that's a giant success for them. It's a great pleasure to be involved in the lives of people who are working hard to keep their chins up and keep moving forward in spite of difficulties. They can be so very inspirational. Here are a few of our favorites.

BABY PAUL

Little Paul was born with a metabolic disorder that caused him to be totally blind. His mother scheduled regular chiropractic treatments to give his little body the best possible chance for normal development. One day after completing his session of cervical release therapy at our office, Mama and Paul were driving back home. Moments later she returned to the clinic with tears of joy in her eyes to share that, as she was driving, Paul was staring sightlessly out the window from the back seat of her car as usual and for the first time his eyes began to squint and then open in response to the sunshine on his face. Although Paul could not speak words of explanation or gratitude, we presume that a bit of his vision had been restored and gave thanks to God for our very small but incredibly welcome success.

MY YOUNG JOSEPHS

I met little Joseph in his second-grade year; he had been diagnosed with severe autism. He started and continued regular chiropractic treatments at our office for many years because his teachers always reported that his ability to concentrate and his communication skills greatly improved as a result of our care. Joseph's enhanced ability to perform was a wonderful win.

I have another patient named Joseph whom I have had the pleasure of treating since he was very young. He is now in 9th grade. This charmer was born with dwarfism. In spite of this sort of "obstacle" Joseph has been a competitive swimmer for most of his life. Even though he is somewhat trapped in a short body, he has grown to be such a giant as he positively impacts the world around him.

VANESSA

While Vanessa is now in her 50s, she could still win a beauty pageant hands down. She is a pastor's wife and the mother of 19-year-old twins. From an outsider's perspective, Vanessa looks as if she has the perfect life. However, unbeknownst to many, she was diagnosed with Multiple Sclerosis almost 20 years ago. Vanessa seeks regular treatments in our clinic to slow the degenerative process of her debilitating disease and to maintain her musculoskeletal health as much as possible.

STEVE

Another of our favorite patients is my dear friend, Steve Bielman. Steve was diagnosed with Primary Lateral Sclerosis or PLS. Like Amyotrophic Lateral Sclerosis (ALS, aka Lou Gehrig's disease), it is a rare progressive neurodegenerative condition. At the time of diagnosis, Steve was a handsome, successful businessman in his 50s. He is married with two wonderful kids. In spite of an otherwise healthy lifestyle, doctors told him that within a short time he would likely be bound to a wheelchair permanently. After more than five years, Steve still drives himself to our clinic in his VW jeep that looks like a fugitive from the hippie era. He comes in smiling and will happily tell the joke of the day to anyone who will listen. Since his PLS condition is advancing more slowly than most documented cases ever, Steve travels all over the country to be studied by many major teaching hospitals. At each station, Steve attributes his success to a clean diet with supplementation, an aggressive fitness program, and regular chiropractic care. He has arrived for treatment in our clinic once a week for many years now, and brings enormous encouragement to everyone he meets.

INFERTILITY

In my office, we love helping couples who are struggling with infertility. When I first met my husband, Tom, I was excited to learn that he already had a notable appreciation for my occupation. He told me that many years before, his parents (Alice and Joe) had grown desperate because they couldn't seem to conceive a child. Alice's friend suggested that she see her chiropractor, who could "solve just about anything". Sure enough, upon evaluation, the chiropractor said that Alice had some displacement in her lumbar spine associated with the nerves linked to her pelvic organs. Alice agreed to a series of chiropractic treatments which did improve her fertility. Over the next 11 years, she gave birth to five children, including my handsome husband, Tom.

ANNIE, MOTHER OF FIVE

My son's second-grade teacher, Annie, came to me for a shoulder problem. She had been on fertility medication for much of her 10-year marriage. Like Alice, her spinal evaluation showed displacement in her lumbar region; so I said that chiropractic adjustment might help. Annie told me that she and her husband were already making arrangements to adopt children. Nevertheless, we treated Annie for the next few weeks.

It was shortly after her first visit that Annie and Steve had the opportunity to adopt two young children whose parents had been killed in an auto accident. Without hesitation, they agreed to take these sweet orphans and began their new family.

The following month I received a call from Annie who giggled unabashedly when she told me that her pregnancy test was finally positive. Annie is convinced that her newfound fertility is the result of her visits to our clinic. Steve and Annie went from having no children to having FIVE young-sters under the age of five. Annie's fertility drugs finally kicked in, helping her to bring forth darling little triplets.

It is not uncommon to find that chiropractic care can help with many cases of infertility. Sometimes, however, we do have to look further than the spine to diagnose the problem. In this case, one of my favorite places is the Jocelyn Center for Natural Fertility. Here they have a 75% success rate of helping women over the age of 40 who have been diagnosed as infertile. That's pretty amazing, compared to our 26% success rate here in the U.S. using radically "unnatural methods" like *in vitro*. Sadly for us, the Jocelyn Center for Natural Fertility is located in Sydney Australia, but I had the fortunate opportunity to study with one of their physicians while she was in Orlando. So at River Hills Clinic, after we have eliminated any spinal displacement components to infertility we look into body chemistry and function. This requires balancing hormones, charting cycles, detoxing mom and dad, and adding supplements with specific nutrients as well as fertility-promoting herbs. An interesting statistic is that 65% of infertility is a male issue so we like to include both partners in our work ups.

MOTHERS AND BABIES

Most gynecologists and obstetricians recommend chiropractic care along with maternity. Many pregnant women suffer some sort of back pain from the altered weight-bearing balance associated with adding the usual 30 extra pounds to their abdomen. Going to the chiropractor for their aches and pains is a much safer solution than medication for both mother and baby. In addition, a properly positioned and properly mobilized pelvis can significantly contribute to the ease of delivery.

Besides helping to position the mother's pelvis, chiropractors can also help to facilitate proper positioning of the unborn baby. Mia, who was nine months pregnant with her seventh child, recently came into our clinic for the special "Webster" chiropractic technique that helps to turn breech babies. After only a couple of treatments, I am happy to report that baby Sarah Grace was in the proper head-down position for her birthday.

Regarding birthing babies, I was introduced to the home birth movement in Atlanta in 1985. It seems we have turned a very old and all-natural process into a high-tech complication which I had never taken much time to evaluate until I became pregnant with my first child. My father-in-law always proudly quoted that all of the U.S. presidents before Jimmy Carter were born at home. When I attended my first home birth meeting, I expected to find a bunch of rebellious hippies in tie-dyed tee shirts with unshaven legs and armpits. Instead, I was surprised to find intelligent professionals who were concerned about exposing their infants to hospital-borne pathogens and wanted to avoid unnecessary medical interventions common in hospital births.

With this prompt, my husband and I chose to birth all four of our sons at home with the assistance of a trained midwife. It was a wonderful experience every time. It seems that my husband proudly shares the stories more often than I do. The most notable was going into labor with my last son while I was still seeing patients at my clinic. I worked hard to stay calm and quiet about the situation so as to not panic anyone or cause a commotion. As the last person left, I sat down at my desk to regroup. Shortly after this, my husband came to check on me and Caleb Michael was born three hours later. My father-in-law did in fact join us for the birth of all four of our sons and actually cut the umbilical cord at the birth of our first; so we named Zachary Joseph after Papa Joe.

YES—CHIROPRACTIC CARE FOR THE EARS

So we do try to adjust pregnant women all the way to their delivery date and later check the spines of their children. Sometimes forceps or plunger-type extraction equipment or other aggressive birthing procedures can cause irritation to a newborn's spine from the very first day, which can impact their future development. The most common reason parents bring their already born babies to a chiropractor is to help resolve chronic ear infections. If a baby's head is not positioned correctly on the neck, it can contribute to a backup of drainage from the estuation tubes. This can cause pressure on the ear drums from the extra fluid and eventually become infected.

Such was the case of baby Fletcher, who suffered with ear infections for much of his first two years of life. The prescribed rounds of antibiotics seemed less effective each time. Finally, the pediatrician recommended surgical implant of drainage tubes in his ear drums. Mom had heard that chiropractic care could possibly help and so she called our clinic for evaluation and treatment of her son. After only a few specific chiropractic adjustments, Fletcher was able to avoid the aggressive intervention and maintain healthy ears ever since. I have continued to take care of Fletcher for most of his life and I am happy to report that he has graduated with honors and is now heading to med school.

SCOLIOSIS SCREENING

Another common reason parents take their children to the chiropractor is for the diagnosis and treatment of scoliosis. For several years our office hosted KID'S DAY AMERICA. This is a nationwide movement of health fairs to promote children's health, safety, and environmental awareness. In addition, River Hills Clinic happily provides the standard scoliosis screening to many of the nearby schools. I think this is so important, and it reminds me of a poster we have that says, *"As a twig is bent so grows the tree."* Skylar was a young man in middle school who was diagnosed with severe scoliosis. His parents brought him to our clinic for a second opinion when it was recommended that he have metal rods surgically implanted into his back to correct the unwanted curvature. Skylar was terrified of this procedure because he knew of another young man who had this procedure done and he could never surf again. (Not good for a Florida boy.) We were delighted when the family chose to follow through with our recommended treatment program and even more delighted when followup x-rays the next year revealed the scoliosis angle was decreased by 28 degrees.

CHIROPRACTIC FOR ATHLETES

After God in his infinite humor blessed my husband and me with our four baby boys, I found myself thrown into the world of little league which appeared to be a permanent fixture. Consequently, I went back to school to pursue yet another specialty and receive my title as a Certified Chiropractic Sports Physician. At the time, I also had the pleasure and privilege of treating a young man named Rex, who was on the Florida Olympic swim team. He made his mom drive him to the clinic for a "spinal tune up" before almost every competition as though it were his lucky rabbit's foot. That year, the Olympics were to be held in Atlanta, and he asked if I could join him if he were to actually make the final cut. The additional certification as a sports physician was necessary to participate as an adjunct physician for Olympic Games so I was happy and hopeful to go the extra mile. In the end, we didn't quite make it to the Olympics but it was fun dreaming together.

So in addition to scoliosis screening in the middle schools, River Hills Clinic also functions as the "Team Chiropractor" for five of the nearby high schools. We tend to many of their sports-related injuries and offer lectures on nutrition, hydration, and conditioning to the players. Every Friday night, we select the "Player of the week" for each team. The winner receives a POTW tee shirt and gets his or her name posted on our website. A little recognition goes a long way.

I love the character development that comes with children playing on sports teams. All four of my sons participated in tee-ball, soccer, wrestling, and football. Their favorite coach was Art Mosley, who always emphasized that integrity and sportsmanship was more important than winning. However, during training, this same coach would shout instructions to, "Run until you throw up!" It seems to me that "Run until you throw up" means you have pushed yourself just about to your physical limitations. I often think about how seldom we actually have the opportunity to push ourselves to our limits to become all that we can be, to "Run until we throw up." Sadly, a lot of times we simply wallow in mediocrity, never knowing what could have been had we truly given our very best.

I'm so proud to share that my son, Matthew, went on to play Division 1 NCAA college football by scholarship. And three of my four sons were part of the Florida State wrestling team and participated and placed in several national tournaments. I owe a lot of their success to exercise, good nutrition, and chiropractic adjustments. Fast forward a few years to brag about my children. I am proud to share that Zachary is now an electronics and social media techy. He is also an entrepreneur in the music world with his own line of clothing. Matthew now lives and works in Phoenix, Arizona. Jordan served in the U.S. Army as an intelligence analyst. Caleb is now seeking a degree in Nutrition and Functional Medicine from the University of Miami.

I love my job which enables people to have their best working body for whatever their purpose and personal assignment is. Our patient, Aaron, plays the French horn for the Jacksonville Symphony Orchestra, Melody is a harp player, Rosanna is an artist, Kevin is a golf pro, Tawambi played football for the Jacksonville Jaguars and the Seattle Sea Hawks, Bob was my Blue Angel Pilot, Albert is my Pearl Harbor survivor, Emily and Megan are our Hollywood actresses, Kristy is a fire-fighter, Kelly is a dancer, Lori is an attorney, Amy is a writer, Larry is a police officer, Brianna is a singer and Jason is a chef. All of these people seek chiropractic care at our clinic to stay on their "A" game.

CHIROPRACTIC FOR SENIORS

We also have special programs for seniors, who gain so much vitality with regular treatment. My friend and patient, Larry Rogers, is a truck driver. He is determined to stay as healthy as he can to work as long as he can. He has attended our yoga and Pilates classes and received chiropractic adjustments for many years now. He plans on living to be 100 and takes every proactive and preventative health care measure that he can to get there. Larry will be 70 in a few months, and he continues to be one of the top performers in our fitness classes. I wish more people would embrace the challenge of aging with as much enthusiasm as Larry does.

Sadly there are so many who chalk up their progressively worsening aches and pains to "old age" long before it's true. In 1986, in Atlanta, Georgia, the wonderful actor, performer, and humanitarian, Bob Hope spoke at my college graduation. He jokingly said, "At my age, my back goes out more often than I do." He lived 17 more years to be 100 years old. If you are sick and tired of being sick and tired, with just a little bit of effort, there are often cures right at your fingertips.

Catherine was another senior patient who was seeking evaluation and treatment for her long-standing neck pain and frozen shoulder. She was a classic slow moving, hunched over little old lady, who could barely move her right arm. We are always happy to see these folks in the clinic because it almost doesn't matter what we do for them, they will probably feel at least a little better, if not a lot better, following their care because they have nowhere to go but up. When Catherine was late for her second visit, the staff and I were concerned that perhaps something we said or did on her first day didn't agree with her or that perhaps something more serious had happened to cause her delay. We were unable to contact her by phone and went on with the afternoon patients. Finally, about two hours later, Catherine showed up beaming from ear to ear. She apologized for being late and explained that when she was taking her shower and getting ready for her appointment that day she was surprised to find that, thanks to her first treatment, she was able to raise her arm enough to do her own hair for the first time in many years. She stayed parked in front of her bathroom mirror for the next hour to "pretty herself up" so as to show her appreciation for our care and her little miracle. People like Catherine keep me smiling for days. Sweet Lillian is the oldest patient I have adjusted. She was 98 when she stopped driving herself to our clinic and moved away to a retirement community.

Musculoskeletal health and staying active is so crucial to our seniors. I am on the Advisory Board for the YMCA. Here we have a whole department of programs called "Silver Sneakers" to focus on this. Sometimes knees and hips get so "worn out" that getting on and off the floor to do exercise is prohibitive. In this case, I always encourage my patients to participate in chair yoga, which allows a significant amount of stretching with the stability of sitting in a chair. If you don't have a YMCA close by, you can get a chair yoga DVD off the internet and do your exercise at home. There is another series of DVDs I love that came out a few years ago to which my mom introduced me. It's called "Walk Away the Pounds". These combine stretching with a good cardio work out and use hand weights, all without having to sit or lie on the floor. So you can kill a bunch of birds with one stone again without ever leaving your house.

Besides the Advisory Board for the YMCA, I am also on The Mayor's Council on Fitness and Well Being. This is a group of 20 local health care professionals who gather monthly to brainstorm and create policies and programs that will improve the health and fitness of our citizens. Our current project is seeking to assign and award Jacksonville as a "Let's Move City". This is an initiative started to tackle the obesity epidemic sweeping America, again focusing on staying active. If you want to live to be a hundred and feel good doing it, if you want to get the most miles out of your body, if you want to perform as efficiently as possible both physically and mentally, you simply must include chiropractic care and spinal checkups in your ongoing health care plan. There are no short cuts. Do you wanna just survive or do you wanna thrive?

COMING FULL CIRCLE

For me, even though it requires more effort to keep up with my middle-aged body, I do enjoy being "older and wiser". A lot has transpired over the years. When I began this career, there was about a 90/10 ratio of male-to-female practitioners. Now there is a 60/40 ratio. I am proud to share that my hearing-impaired little brother is now six feet tall. He paddled against the current to finish school and grew up to become a wonderful man. He is a sign language interpreter and instructor. David has worked and studied his way to being a high-level minister in his church congregation. He lights a candle in the darkness at every opportunity he can find.

I was recently assigned to be the liaison between the Mayo Clinic and our local chiropractic community. It's interesting that with all of Mayo's amazing physicians and amazing diagnostic equipment that the smartest and first round of defense against

151

disease and aging is still going back to the basics. Losing sight of the basics has increased the need for hospital care. There's a sign in my office that says: "If you wear out your body, where are you gonna live?"

The two biggest factors contributing to vitality and longevity are, in fact, diet and lifestyle. This is such good news because you can do a lot to contribute to that, whether it is getting regular spinal checkups at your chiropractor, or making healthier food choices, getting better sleep, increasing your physical activity, or decreasing the stress in your life. Another factor contributing to your health profile is your genetic makeup, but it's a distant third. This you can't do much to change your genetics but you can educate yourself in ways to efficiently manage the weaknesses you have been dealt. My son, who played college football, is actually a type one (Juvenile) Diabetic. I was born with a heart defect which required an open heart surgery when I was an infant. This was at the University of Michigan in a time that these procedures were not very developed. The doctors told my parents that I had less than 50/50 chance of survival and here I am 50+ years later. Always remember that, in spite of what it looks like, God has a very important purpose for your life. You simply do the best you can with what you've got.

AN ANCIENT ILLUSTRATION

A while back, I heard an illustration from a pastor that left a permanent impact in my life and on my practice. His message came in three parts.

First, he reminded us of the Bible story of Martha and Mary. These were Jesus's close friends. During His travels, He stopped by their home for food and lodging. Mary sat at Jesus's feet in order to absorb His every word and gesture. Martha spent the time busying herself with necessary kitchen preparations and missed the special opportunity to bask in His holiness. To me, this lesson reminds us to keep our priorities straight. People are more important than things. It can be difficult to balance all of the details and responsibilities of our lives but I think that "everything in moderation" applies very often.

The second part of Pastor Brett's illustration was the day when Martha and Mary sent a messenger to Jesus, who was in a nearby city, asking Him to come quickly to heal their brother Lazarus from a deathly illness. Most of us remember the very unusual response: HE DIDN'T COME.

Even though Martha, Mary, and Lazarus were very close friends of Jesus, HE DIDN'T COME. Lazarus died. The Biblical account of this incident relates that several days after Lazarus was entombed, Jesus finally DID come. I assume that the sisters were probably sad, maybe angry, and almost certainly very confused. In the times of our worst stress and confusion, we should remind ourselves that God is obviously smarter than we are and really does know what is in our best interest.

Jesus went on to actually RAISE LAZARUS FROM THE DEAD. Perhaps Jesus was thinking that if He wanted to display God's love and mighty strength to that community, raising a person from the dead would leave a greater impact than simply bringing a tissue to wipe away sniffles.

So I share this illustration with friends, colleagues, and patients alike. When life throws us one of those unexpected curve balls, remember that God is still in control, and can make good things come from very bad experiences. No one escapes heartbreak and overwhelming obstacles. Live, love, learn, and keep moving forward.

The third part of this illustration is specifically for doctors taking care of their patients, and for patients who take care of their friends and families. This story ends when Jesus asks Martha and Mary to take him to the tomb that held Lazarus' dead body. Both of the girls were hesitant to go—perhaps they wanted to avoid the horrific sight and smell of a decomposing body. Still Jesus insisted. When they arrived at the tomb with Lazarus' mourning friends and family, Jesus simply said, "Lazarus—come forth!"

At this point, Jesus could have made Lazarus appear before them, alive, and dressed in a glorious silk robe. Instead, the Bible tells us that Lazarus rose alive and presented himself wrapped in the unflattering mummy-looking strips of cloth in which dead bodies were customarily bound. It was then that Jesus said the most wonderful words of all: "UNBIND HIM!"

This is another message that we can carry with us through life. God could, in fact, solve all of the big and small problems that we encounter, but He prefers to use us to minister to one another. "Unbind him!" He tells us to unbind those around us, whether physically or mentally or spiritually. I take these instructions very seriously and do my best to facilitate those around me to do the same for the people around them.

So I say to all of my past, present, and future friends and patients: it has been such an honor and a privilege to be part of your health care team. We will do everything we can to help you live happier, healthier, longer lives.

With much love and gratitude—KEEP SHINING!

(This content should be used for informational purposes only. It does not create a doctor-patient relationship with any reader and should not be construed as medical advice. If you need medical advice, please contact a doctor in your community who can assess the specifics of your situation.)

7

HEADACHES - THEY'RE NOT ALL IN YOUR HEAD

by Kenneth A. Frank, D.C.

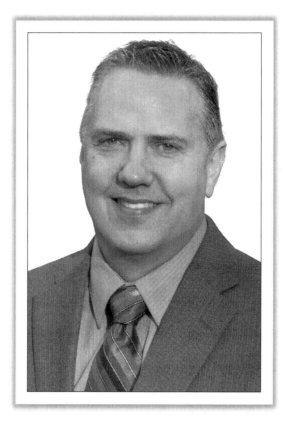

Kenneth A. Frank, D.C.

Kenneth A. Frank, D.C. Chiropractic
Folsom, California
www.kennethfrankdc.com

Dr. Frank is passionate about the healing and education of his patients. His services are encompassed under the umbrella of Neuro-Metabolic care, which is the blending of the best of Brain Based Therapies, Clinical Nutrition, and Spinal Corrective Care. He has a doctorate in Chiropractic and is a California board certified Chiropractor.

Dr. Frank was trained in Chiropractic Neurology by Dr. John Donofrio, President of the American Chiropractic Neurology Board. He was trained in Clinical Nutrition, in Head Trauma and Brain Injuries, in Professional Development by Regent University. He is trained in Neurological Brain Based Therapy, specializing in treating chronic conditions, chronic pain, neurological and autoimmune conditions with emphasis on migraines and chronic headaches. His techniques are neurologically specific adjustment techniques, pneumatic air insufflation technique, interferential therapy, trigger point therapy, proprioceptive neuromuscular facilitation technique, Gonstead technique, Diversified technique, and Activator technique.

HEADACHES - THEY'RE NOT ALL IN YOUR HEAD

I get a lot of satisfaction from helping people and I am especially passionate about helping folks with migraines because my wife used to suffer from them. "Brain Based Therapy" is the newest cutting-edge breakthrough treatment for migraines, chronic headaches, and many other conditions. I will discuss several conditions and how a combination of Brain Based Therapy, Clinical Nutrition, and Spinal Corrective Care are key components in achieving the best outcome. This integrative comprehensive approach allows me to see and understand what's "really" causing a patient's symptoms so that I can give them a specific customized treatment plan.

MIGRAINE HEADACHES

I work a lot with migraine patients and consider treating them one of my specialties. It's very satisfying to help people with this debilitating condition. I need to understand the "WHY" of a persons headache before I can treat them effectively. By unraveling the mystery, I can develop a specific plan that works for them. There are many possible causes of migraines and chronic headaches, however, in my practice I have found several underlying causes that need to be addressed to adequately treat chronic migrane and headache conditions.

Essentially, one underlying cause of migraines is a brain weakness or a brain imbalance (hemisphericity). Commonly, a person with this condition has a part of their brain that isn't as strong as the other parts. In many cases, the weak section is the cerebellum (back part of the brain). When I say weak, I mean that the nerve signals from that side of the cerebellum are not firing at the frequency they are supposed to. The body is designed to be in balance; problems occur when there is an imbalance.

A looping connection forms as the cerebellum fires signals to the frontal lobe, and the frontal lobe sends signals to the brainstem. If the cerebellum is weak and not firing appropriately, then you have lost that essential looping connection. Remember, your brain is communicating to the tissues, bones, and even the individual cells within your body, and your body provides feedback to the brain. When this loop breaks down, so can your health.

When the cerebellum isn't firing appropriately, the upper brainstem (mesencephalon) overfires and puts your system into fight or flight mode (sympathetic nervous system activates). As a result, the blood vessels in your brain expand. Your blood vessels are sheathed in pain fibers, so when the blood vessels expand more than usual, as in this case, the pain fibers get stretched. You experience that expansion as pain. This sensation of pain is also known as a "vascular headache".

In a classic migraine, the cranial nerves arising - from the brainstem, that link to different areas of the head and face, are over-excited. One of the affected nerves, the "oculomotor nerve," controls the functions of your eyes. When the oculomotor nerve becomes over-stimulated, the pupils widen to let more light in. This is why unfortunate migraine sufferers are sensitive to light and have to lie down in the dark.

Another important nerve, called the "vagus nerve", is acranial nerve that comes out of the brainstem. The vagus nerve wanders all over your body, but it also reaches down to your gut. When that nerve has been over-stimulated, the patient will experience nausea, sometimes to the point of vomiting.

New research tells us that there's another factor called "cortical spreading depression" (CSD). In migraines, neurologists have found that there is a wave of activity in the cortex of the brain that relates to the expansion and contraction of the blood vessels and the oxygen supply to the brain. This wave travels through the cortex and seems to be associated with the scintillating scotoma, that visual "aura" that sometimes precedes a migraine. The latest research suggests that a thorough neurological evaluation is indicated so that doctors can evaluate your brain, spinal cord, and nerves. In order to solve the problem, they must discover which part of the brain is not working correctly.

Courtesy of Dr. Frederick Robert "Ted" Carrick, comes the new revolutionary treatment called "Brain-Based Therapy," an effective option. Dr. Carrick is the top chiropractic neurologist in the country and he is responsible for this incredible work. Doctor Carrick has developed an all-natural therapy for migraines, chronic headaches and many other conditions. It's accomplished through simple yet powerful exercises and therapies.

CHIROPRACTIC ADJUSTMENTS & HEADACHES

Another underlying cause of headaches is a cervicogenic problem, which means that it originates in the cervical spine (neck), usually around the upper vertebrae in the neck which surrounds the brainstem from which the cranial nerves emerge. We address this cause with chiropractic treatment. When there's a specific misalignment of the upper neck, we realign that area, taking the pressure off the brainstem, and that will generally help with most headaches.

These days, many people have a loss of neck curvature caused by continually looking down. Since people use so many technological items (computers or mobile phones for texting) that require them to look down or constantly bend their heads forward, this position can create difficulty over time. If this situation stretches on for months or years, people start to lose the curve in their necks. In turn, this curve loss puts pressure on the brainstem and becomes a pain in the head, also known as a headache. Chiropractic spinal corrective care and neck adjustments will help with the pain.

I also help my patients with a few other helpful adjustments, including a rib adjustment and unilateral (one sided) adjustments. The rib adjustment will help to loosen up that area and relax the muscles around the ribcage and thoracic spine (mid-back). That simple relaxation will also help with easing headaches. For quick results with migraines, our office also uses a technique that's relatively new called "pneumatic air insufflation technique." We use an insufflation bulb to blow air gently into the ear canal at certain frequencies. This works amazingly well at promptly reducing or eliminating the headache in the office. This alone is not a cure because it does not address the underlying cause, however patients really appreciate it. The overall brain treatment takes some time, but for someone suffering through a migraine, the air insufflation can provide quick relief.

Another thing to keep in mind is, if you overuse headache medicine (Advil,Tylenol etc.), it may cause rebound headaches.

STRESS AND HEADACHES

As I tell my patients with chronic pain and headaches, you cannot ignore the key role of stress in all of these issues and conditions, since stress affects your brain, internal organs and muscles. Here, I am talking about "emotional stress". When your sympathetic nervous system kicks in to assist with the "fight or flight" response (discussed earlier), your muscles contract and tighten up. Your body then pumps extra blood to the extremities that will be most necessary in handling the crisis. All of that activity creates a diversion of the blood flow and the resulting amounts of oxygen flow. As you have more blood and oxygen flowing through your muscles, your brain and internal organs are not getting their usual supply of oxygen and blood. Over time, your internal system will break down. So, if you're stressed more than just once in a while, it can lead to conditions such as: chronic fatigue syndrome, fibromyalgia, depression and insomnia, thyroid problems, obesity, irritable bowel syndrome (IBS), gerd (gastro-esophageal reflux disease),ulcers, ulcerative colitis, chron's disease, leaky gut syndrome, reproductive issues, and autoimmune conditions.

When you can get the muscles to relax, more blood flow and more oxygen flows through the tissues and into the brain. You will begin to feel better and your headaches will improve if you can catch it right away. That's what happens with the rib adjustment, which keeps the biomechanics (movement) of the ribcage moving properly, thus allowing full inspiration and expiration, getting more oxygen to flow to your brain.

In this modern age of stress, we all know about and understand physical and emotional stress. However, there's also something called "chemical stress", related to items such as artificial sweeteners. Aspartame (NutraSweet and Equal), Sucralose (Splenda), and other artificial sweeteners act as poison to the body. These chemicals are toxins to the nervous system and to the brain, and will cause a brain weakness and imbalance.

THE BRAIN/GUT CONNECTION

Inflammation of the brain tissue is another underlying cause of migraines and chronic headaches. This means the brain is literally inflamed, which means it's not working right. Interestingly, research shows that the brain and gut are connected, so in discussing the brain, you're also talking about the gut, where your immune system "lives". So, the brain controls the gut, and the gut controls the immune system. Finally, the immune system sends back reports to the brain. If there is any break in the completion of that loop you have a problem.

So, how do people develop inflammation in the brain? If a person's system is overloaded by a bad diet and toxins, such as food allergens/sensitivities, gluten or genetically modified organisms (GMOs), these can affect the gut and cause inflammation. Remember, the brain and the gut are completely connected.

In my office, we begin the entire inflammatory review process with an overall nutritional assessment, which essentially gives us a snapshot of the body and all of the systems within it. We take a long look at the digestive system—the gut—and review the activity happening inside of it. Migraine sufferers and chronic headache sufferers will have digestive gut issues. Through nutritional intervention, we work to reduce both the gut and brain inflammation by changing the diet and using nutritional protocols.

As chiropractors, when we're trying to help a patient with headaches or any other kind of problem, the use of these toxins counteracts our efforts. Antibiotics, corticosteroids (prednisone) and NSAIDS (Advil , Aleve), will also kill and damage the important flora in the intestines. I've already explained that the gut is connected to the brain in a continual loop, so if one of my patient's takes antibiotics, she is not only going to have a gut problem, she's going to have a brain imbalance. By the way, approximately 70 percent of our immune system is in our gut.

Where there's inflammation, there's a loss of function—things don't work correctly. Inflammation is your body's way of taking a part of the body out of the game. For example, twisting your ankle causes it to become inflamed, and you can't walk on it without pain. When you experience gut inflammation, brain inflammation is also taking place.

Many of us have poor eating habits, causing many problems in the gut and, therefore, in the brain. You might experience symptoms such as mental fog, sluggish thinking, and/or blurry vision. Common triggers for these symptoms include wheat, barley, rye, corn and spelt as well as dairy products. Soy can create difficulties, as can the more obvious triggers like processed sugar, high fructose corn syrup, and white salt. (Look for pink salt.)

Many patients are in need of a detoxification protocol to handle their chemical stress. The system assessment form will help me identify these patients. If your system is clogged, both the liver and gallbladder will show signs and symptoms. If the patient has digestive problems, he or she is going to need a detox/purification program to get rid of that buildup in order to make significant progress.

Since another underlying cause may be related to "Food Sensitivities", we can order specific lab tests if we suspect that there are allergens associated with certain foods. Another way to uncover the culprit(s) is to start eliminating common allergens and observe and monitor the patient's reactions and symptoms. Hormonal changes and imbalances can be another underlying cause of migraines or chronic headaches. We will need to figure out the specific nutritional protocol that will help to balance the hormones.

Another cause of headaches can be traced to those substances that you *don't* ingest. Dehydration can cause chronic headaches. Drinking half of your body weight in ounces every day is recommended. If you weigh 150 pounds, you need to put 75 ounces of water in your body every day. Water is very important.

GASTROINTESTINAL COMPLAINTS

For patients with a gastrointestinal complaint, the first thing that I do is take a look at my patient's brain to get an overall picture of its activity (refer to gut-brain connection earlier in the chapter). This is accomplished by doing a thorough neurological evaluation. As most of us have experienced when we're under stress or nervous about something, the stomach is almost always upset and churning. Everybody can relate to that particular connection. Most of us have also noticed that certain foods alter our moods, focus or con-centration. Essentially, I'm often dealing with a brain imbalance that's compounded by what my patient is putting into his or her system. This may be a familiar idea, but we, as people, need to eat more carefully and be more selective about what we put into our bodies.

If I find a problem in my client's GI system, my first step is to move toward healing and balancing out the GI tract, recognizing that he or she may have "Leaky Gut Syndrome". Specific nutritional protocols are used to heal the intestinal lining, then seal it up. Medical doctors recognize this condition, but they sometimes call it a mystery. If you look this condition up online at one of the medical encyclopedia sites like WebMD, you'll find that the medical science community doesn't thoroughly understand the problem.

The symptoms of leaky gut syndrome consist of bloating, gas, cramps, food sensitivities, fatigue , eczema , migraines, diarrhea, constipation, brain fog and general aches and pains. Many people with leaky gut syndrome, however, have no intestinal or inflammatory symptoms, especially if they already eat a healthy diet with limited pro-inflammatory foods. So, leaky gut should be considered for anyone with brain fog, persistent depression, chronic systemic inflammation, or any autoimmune condition, even if you don't have digestive symptoms. When this group of symptoms presents itself, I begin by evaluating the nutritional aspect of my patient's life, because these symptoms can be triggered by unnatural substances like: antibiotics (anti = against bio= life), NSAIDS (Advil, Aleve), as well as food allergens, gmo's, emotional stress, gluten, bacteria, parasites or yeast. In general, and over time, these things will begin to affect the lining of your intestines. Your intestines have a barrier that is designed to pull nutrients out of your food and into your bloodstream so that you can use them as fuel and then remove the other items to be discharged as waste.

"Autoimmune Conditions" develop after the gut lining becomes compromised. When foreign objects (yeast, bacteria, viruses, parasites) enter the bloodstream because of the damaged, porous lining, your immune system simply recognizes invaders. When foreign bodies invade the immune system, its job is to act like Pac-Man (scavengers): attack them, beat them up, and dispose of the whole bunch. For example, if the foreign bodies are lodged in the thyroid gland, you end up with an inflammation of the thyroid gland while the battle rages. If the toxins appear in a different organ or system, that's where the inflammation and problem will occur. That's why your immune system sometimes attacks your own body. So called incurable diseases with unknown causes are caused by this mechanism, where the body attacks its own system.

In thyroid-related issues, my practice has found that 90 percent of those cases are accompanied by gut problems.

BRAIN BASED THERAPY – THE MISSING LINK

Brain Based Therapy (BBT) is a revolutionary new treatment for previously difficult to treat problems such as migraines, vertigo, dizziness and balance disorders, sciatica, fibromyalgia, chronic fatigue, irritable bowel syndrome, thyroid disorders, insomnia and many other chronic conditions. Based on the work of Chiropractic Neurologist Dr. Ted Carrick, this new treatment uses our understanding of the human brain, its controlling influence over all other body systems, the ways that it loses its optimal "frequency of firing" and the many health problems that result.

Through specialized tests, I am able to pinpoint the area(s) of energy deficit in the brain. With a combination of neurological treatments and chiropractic techniques it's then possible to target and recharge the depleted-weak areas. This fixes the cause of the problem and provides relief from pain and other chronic symptoms that pills and ordinary treatment procedures cannot.

Keep in mind, there are two types of brain issues, hard and soft. Hard lesions are things like multiple sclerosis, strokes or tumors. I address soft lesions primarily, which deal with imbalances of the brain. I am trained in functional neurology and do a very thorough neurological exam to pinpoint the problem area of the brain. The good news is that the soft lesions are correctable!

Science has shown that the brain is plastic and adaptable, so to speak. The brain has the ability to form new nerve connections. This is called neuroplasticity. The brain can be strengthened just as a muscle can be built up for better performance. The weak part of a brain can be strengthened and brought into balance with the stronger side, thus restoring the brain's equilibrium, which is the ultimate goal of the body. If you have this condition, it doesn't necessarily mean that the brain weakness will show up in memory loss issues, nor does it mean that you're just stuck with that weakness. Again, there is hope because this is fixable.

This research comes from multiple fields of medicine: psychology, neurology, neurophysiology, and nutrition. Each discipline plays a part. Using neurological evaluation and brain evaluation, I locate the area of weakness. Once we know where the weakness lies, we do therapeutic work in the office and also give home exercises to the patient to be done outside the office. We customize brain therapies to increase the firing of that weaker part of the brain, so that the two sides eventually become synchronized.

A unilateral (one sided) adjustment is one of the examples of brain therapies used in my office. Put simply, we adjust the spine and extremities on one side only to fire muscle receptors and joint mechanoreceptors (joint receptors) into the opposite cerebral cortex (brain). The mid-back will be globally manipulated to fire the dorsal columns (back part of the spinal cord) and reduce rib fixations. The left side of the brain controls the right side of the body and vice versa, so we do our work on the opposite side of the body to help the weaker side of the brain.

We also do eye exercises and auditory stimulation that involve playing music into just one ear of our patient. Eye exercises are used to increase the frequency of firing of the cerebellum (back part of the brain). We also add in aromatherapy, arm swing therapy, and spin therapy. These activities, in time, will exercise and serve to strengthen the side of the brain that needs strength training. Additionally, there are deep breathing exercises to increase the oxygen flow to the brain.

SCIATICA?

When considering the totality of brain-based therapy, which I think is the missing link in healthcare, it's also important to consider the condition known as *Sciatica*. The sciatic nerve comes out of the lower back and runs all the way down to the bottom of the foot and toes. If the nerve is affected, it will cause pain and other symptoms. Let's say that the patient gets treated or the issue is temporarily fixed, but even though he or she does the suggested stretches and exercises, they still experience a recurring problem. If the problem keeps reappearing, that would suggest a brain imbalance.

Here's how it works. The cerebellum controls the spinal postural muscles as well as balance and coordination. So, if the cerebellum is weak, you will get contracting and pulling on all the spinal muscles on one side or the other. It will pull the vertebrae to that side, lock them in place, or make them stick. That impacts the entire joint, including the disc and everything in that whole joint. In the chiropractic field, our mission is to un-stick the stuck vertebrae. In this situation, even if we do our un-sticking, the vertebrae will constantly be pulled to one side. This joint fixation is called a misalignment or subluxation. There can be no permanent relief because it will constantly be irritating that nerve, due to the fact that there is a weakness or imbalance in the brain that's causing the underlying problem. In other words, Sciatic nerve symptoms and appearances may be caused by a brain imbalance.

In order to permanently resolve the problem, the brain imbalance needs to be fixed, so that the muscles will start relaxing on that one side. Eventually, that whole joint, where the sciatic nerve emerges from the spine, can be coaxed back to normal. That's why I call Brain Based Therapy the "Missing Link" for Sciatica and other conditions—it's not always considered or applied in terms of finding a solution to a recurring or chronic problem.

NEUROLOGICAL COMPLAINTS

We also see neurological complaints associated with the head and face area.

Trigeminal neuralgia (prosopalgia or Fothergill's disease) has also been called the suicide syndrome. "Neuralgia" means "nerve pain". This fairly rare complaint leads to horrible pain in the facial nerves. The pain from the trigeminal nerve, which is one of those nerves that comes out of the brainstem and branches out to the face, can become so intense that those who have that pain want to commit suicide.

I just treated a few people with this type of neuralgia. First, I check the brain to see which side is imbalanced. I know that there's an imbalance because the firing loop includes the trigeminal nerve, which comes out of the brainstem. The mesencephalon (upper brain stem) over-fires and irritates this nerve. The nerve runs down the face and the cheek and jaw area, and the over-activity creates intermittent but intense pain along the cheek. Step one is to start the brain balancing treatment.

Step two includes checking the chewing muscles (masseters). One side will feel a lot tighter than the other. (The same system of treatment will also help with various types of temporomandibular disorders or TMJ.) I use a technique that I call "stripping of the muscle," which involves some muscle manipulation to lessen the friction that occurs between the muscle and the trigeminal nerve. This helps to release that overexcited muscle which is constantly grabbing at the trigeminal nerve.

In step three, I adjust the upper neck because the upper neck surrounds the brainstem. The adjustment will reduce the pressure on the trigeminal nerve. Those three activities are the way in which my office deals with trigeminal neuralgia or even TMJ. Since Tinnitus can have a brain imbalance component, it will also respond to this three-step process. My work as a chiropractor is to calm the nerve that goes to the ear. Later, I find and strengthen the brain to fix my patient's brain imbalance, then I adjust the upper neck.

VERTIGO, DIZZINESS AND BALANCE DISORDERS

Vertigo, dizziness, and other balance problems are usually a brain issue, but these can also be vestibular, which involves the inner-ear. Chiropractic care can help with that to a certain extent, depending upon the circumstances of the case. If a patient is having balance issues, we would do a thorough neurological evaluation to determine hemisphericity. In other words, we determine which hemisphere of the brain is involved. When a problem makes an appearance on one side of the brain or the other, it leads back to an imbalance in the brain.

A thorough neurological evaluation can determine the part of the brain that is weak or poorly firing and is functioning at less than peak levels. When patients show signs of this particular problem, I check the cerebellum. Why? The cerebellum controls your balance, your coordination, and the stability of your postural muscles at the spine. Naturally, the cerebellum is the part of the brain that I suspect when my patient complains of vertigo and dizziness.

At that point, my job is to increase the frequency of firing, thus stimulating that part of the brain, and to increase the nerve impulses so that they are stronger. The good news is that you're not simply stuck with vertigo or memory loss. With a series of special exercises and therapies, we can rebuild the brain, as mentioned earlier in the chapter.

The brain needs two things to stay healthy: fuel and activation. The brain is fueled through glucose. Your body breaks down all of the food you consume into glucose so that you'll have energy to perform all of the functions in the body. The best form of glucose comes in the form of organic whole foods. I recommend specific whole food supplements to the patient, including the foods that feed and nourish the brain, or brain foods. I recommend specific supplements with specific dosages to my patients then monitor them monthly. A few brain nourishing supplements are coconut oil, CoQ10, omega 3 fatty acids, and grape seed.

Oxygen is the other point of focus. Your body will ship oxygen to the brain and the heart without fail. However, if you're not exercising with the involvement of your lungs, you may be experiencing a shortage of oxygen. We prescribe deep breathing exercises to get that oxygen pumping to the brain. Deep breathing should happen on a one-to-two ratio, meaning that you breathe out (exhale) twice as long as the time you take to inhale.

I will also talk to my patients about walking a specified distance per day to increase their oxygen uptake.

The first steps in balancing the brain involve addressing oxygen and glucose. The next step is activation and stimulation. Our revolutionary breakthrough drugless treatment, "Brain-Based Therapy", incorporates simple yet powerful exercises and rehabilitation. Once we determine which side of the brain is weaker, the patient and I work on the functions of the opposite side of the body from that section of the brain, because the brain and body functions are opposite or crisscrossed. Visual stimulation and exercises are used to increase the firing to the cerebellum (back of the brain) and frontal lobe of the brain, as well as auditory stimulation in one ear to stimulate the ipsilateral (same side) cerebellum. We also stimulate the olfactory system on one side in order to strengthen and increase the firing to the same side of the brain and opposite cerebellum.

The last step is the therapeutic component of spinal corrective care. We do chiropractic adjustments to normalize "proprioception", which means the individual's awareness of posture or his sense of balance or position. An adjustment will improve vertigo, dizziness, and balance disorders because it reduces pressure from the brain stem, which also helps to balance the brain. One sided adjustments are done to the spine and extremities to increase the firing and strengthen the same side cerebellum and opposite cerebral cortex (brain).

ATHLETIC IMPLICATIONS

In terms of athletic performance, this kind of treatment program can give an edge to any athlete because the cerebellum controls balance, coordination, and the spinal postural muscles. The cerebellum also controls the individual's proprioception (as discussed in the previous section). By balancing the brain, we can synchronize the parts of the body.

For example, with your brain and both sides of your body communicating at peak levels, you can decrease the number of strokes in your golf game. Synchronization will improve your reflexes and performance in all physical activities, such as improving your shooting percentage in basketball. Additionally, this kind of treatment can also prevent injuries. Instead of spraining your ankle when you take an awkward step, your other ankle muscles will be stronger, better able to protect each other. With your new, improved sense of where you are and how your muscles are placed in relation to the world, the misstep might not happen at all. The bottom line benefits: To give you the edge in any sport or activity that you participate in and to help you prevent injuries.

EXPLANATION OF THE SUBLUXATION AND ADJUSTMENT PROCESS

When patients think of chiropractors, they often think of our common field terms, "subluxation" and "adjustment". I'll try to explain the process of adjustment. Essentially, dysfunction and pain set in due to joint fixation. Cartilage begins to break down into polypeptides, which stimulate nerve cells that detect harm (nociception) in the nervous system and in the brain's sensory and motor control center (thalamus), and on to the limbic system which is then experienced as pain. Also, this causes a reflexive muscle contraction in a scleratogenous distribution, causing pain and spasms. The lack of joint motion causes irregular firing so we get either too much excitation or inhibition which changes the frequency of firing to the brain resulting in an imbalance of information as perceived by the brain that can alter overall neurological motor function.

An adjustment of that subluxation causes the body to start protein replication of DNA, which keeps a negative charge inside the cell, thus preventing neural degeneration and cell death. This improves tissue maintenance and repair throughout the entire system. DNA replication improves inter-cellular communication, which improves overall system function. The adjustment also breaks the fixation component, which inhibits certain nerve receptors from firing at an increased rate therefore decreasing pain and spasm.

THE CHIROPRACTIC SOLUTION

A chiropractic adjustment is a wonderful tool that can give the patient a number of beneficial results.

1. An adjustment can restore motion, including the entire range of motion on both sides.

2. It will normalize your biomechanics and load distribution. The vertebrae work to give you even weight distribution on all vertebrae and joints. You will want to restore symmetry and balance.

3. An adjustment helps to get your body to pump out waste products and edematous fluid. When your vertebrae are misaligned or get stuck, your body creates swelling (edema) in the muscles to keep them from moving. The swelling and inflammation gets released after an appropriate adjustment; the body pumps out extra fluid in the problem area. This allows the joint to move more freely.

4. By improving the motion of the joints, the adjustment can improve the flow of nutrition to the disk and the articular cartilage (cartilage surrounding the joint).

5. An adjustment supports or maintains the health of the vertebrae, joints, and disks, which helps to relax the tight muscles.

6. An adjustment can normalize proprioception (your awareness of posture, balance, and positioning sense).

7. An adjustment stimulates the sensory and motor reflexes, which improve dynamic muscular stabilization of the joints. Going without an adjustment for a period of time leads to weak joints and slower reaction times. An adjustment is a powerful way to enhance the communication between the brain and the joints.

8. Adjustments accelerate healing by increasing blood flow, collagen, and protein production.

9. It ensures the proper alignment of new connective tissue to prevent scarring of the tissues around the joint.

The terrain of the healthcare world is changing and people are reaching out for answers. A key concept I would like to express is that people are people, not conditions. They suffer from conditions but they must be treated as individuals. We treat the body not the disease. You lose if you try to treat the disease, you win if you treat the body.

In my experience, chiropractic care can successfully deal with these problems: vertigo and balance disorders, back and neck pain, dizziness, sciatica, restless leg syndrome, migraines and chronic headaches, numbness and tingling, chronic fatigue, fibromyalgia, thyroid disorders, carpal tunnel syndrome, shoulder problems, brain fog, irritable bowel syndrome, diabetes, high blood pressure, and autoimmune conditions. It's a pretty impressive list.

ONE HAPPY PATIENT

One day, a 45-year old female arrived at the office with a number of issues: joint pain in every joint (arms, legs, etc.), constant migraines, bloating, heartburn, and constipation. She was having only one or two bowel movements per week.

We began a detox/purification program for a few weeks, just to clear all of the toxins and poisons out of her system. Once that was done, we started brain-based therapy and the spinal corrective care. You can't go wrong with that three-pronged approach, which deals with restoring balance and eliminating physical and chemical stressors. The package of treatment makes a huge difference. The patient's constant and severe joint pain completely cleared up, along with most of her migraines. She still gets an occasional migraine, mostly due to eye strain and stress. Even so, there is a significant difference between constant and occasional migraines. Her bloating and heartburn completely disappeared. With treatment, her bowels were moving at a normal rate of one or two times every day, which represents a major difference. As a bonus, she lost approximately 12 pounds. Usually, this program is not intended as a weight-loss program. However, once you detox and purify, the body can remove the toxic sludge and you'll naturally lose some weight. Of course, she is happy about that little side benefit.

As I said in the beginning, my passion and my focus is to help people with migraines and chronic headaches. The approach in my practice goes beyond migraines and chronic headaches to chronic pain, chronic conditions in general, and autoimmune diseases. I treat people neurologically, metabolically and with spinal corrective care. I provide a unique, integrative, holistic approach in getting to the cause of your problem. I support and treat YOU the person, not your symptoms, condition or disease.

(This content should be used for informational purposes only. It does not create a doctor-patient relationship with any reader and should not be construed as medical advice. If you need medical advice, please contact a doctor in your community who can assess the specifics of your situation.)

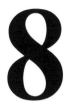

8

HOW MUCH
EXPERIENCE DOES
YOUR CHIROPRACTOR
HAVE?

by Brian D. Reimer, D.C.

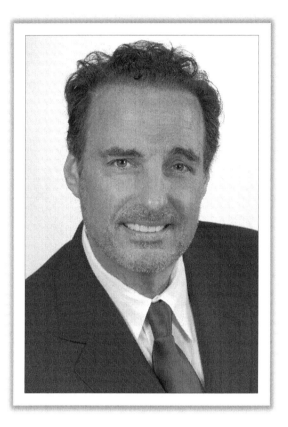

Brian D. Reimer, D.C.
American Med Care
West Palm Beach, Florida
www.chiropractic-westpalmbeach.com

Dr. Brian D. Reimer has been a practicing chiropractor for 35 years. He graduated from Logan Chiropractic College in Chesterfield, MO in 1979. He went on to attain licenses in the states of Missouri, New York, and Florida. Dr. Reimer began practicing in his native New York for one year and moved to beautiful Palm Beach County Florida in 1980 where he practiced and owned multiple chiropractic offices. Dr. Reimer later went on to combine chiropractic and medical care as a multidisciplinary form of healthcare and continues practicing the science, art and philosophy of chiropractic because of his desire to Give, Love and Serve is patients.

He has been an active member of the A.C.A. the F.C.A., and the F.C.P.A., he was an honored member of the Heritage Registry of Who's Who 2007-2008, also listed in the Who's Who Worldwide registry whose members are limited to those individuals who have demonstrated outstanding leadership and achievement in their profession. Dr. Reimer was also listed in the Guide to America's Top Chiropractors under Back and Spine care.

HOW MUCH EXPERIENCE DOES YOUR CHIROPRACTOR HAVE?

I hope to shed some light on what chiropractors do in general and what I do specifically to help my patients live happier, healthier lives with much less pain. Some of you may be familiar with chiropractic care, while others may not. However, after 35 years as a practicing chiropractor, I can tell you that all chiropractic practices are not cut from one mold.

In your search for a chiropractor, you will find some whose focus is totally holistic—they take on nearly any kind of problem. My practice sticks with more traditional musculoskeletal areas and treatments. We primarily deal with the spine, the entire nervous system, and conditions that typically stem from spinal problems: neck pain, back pain, headache, trauma, and injury. We see every kind of trauma-related pain in our practice: work-related injuries, falls, injuries from car accidents, etc. We also treat the kind of pain that patients wake up with one day: back pain, neck pain, shoulder pain, or knee pain. Some patients look for chiropractors to deal with other systemic types of conditions or medical conditions that may not fall under the norm of chiropractic care, which is fine. I just try to excel at what I do without reaching too far beyond the chiropractic foundation.

In choosing a doctor of any kind, but especially a chiropractor, the first thing that you should examine is his level of experience. I believe that the doctor, who has been in practice for a long period of time, with a great deal of experience in recognizing and treating many different conditions, brings with him some important advantages.

Given that premise, the best way for a patient to find chiropractic care is through a personal referral. The best referrals are from somebody you know and trust who has used the doctor and has some personal experience of his techniques and his use of technology. In other words, does he use state-of-the-art tools and techniques? You can use the Internet for this kind of research. The doctor's website will probably tell you which conditions he treats and how he treats them. To begin a search for a chiropractor, two excellent websites are Spine-Health www.spine-health.com or Spine Universe www.spineuniverse.com. If possible, talk to somebody who knows the doctor and his practice.

Additionally, because there is almost always a need for the next step after the basic chiropractic care, find a chiropractor who offers physical therapy in-office. When chiropractors attempt to treat a typical musculoskeletal condition, physical therapy can add another layer of benefit to the offered amount of care.

FOCUS ON THE RESULT YOU WANT

In your search, it's helpful to know what results you actually want to find. What would it take for you to call the process a "success"? Would it be to reduce the pain by 90 percent? How much more, in terms of actual range of motion, would be enough? Our chiropractic care can be great for you, but so much depends upon your condition as well as the results that you want to see. One way to know this is to find a practice that offers a first consultation at no charge.

Our office tries to obtain a good understanding of expectations right up front. If you and the doctor both understand what success looks like, it's easier to conclude whether or not you'll both be satisfied with the result. A patient's particular expectations might not be something that we can provide. I'd much rather tell patients in the beginning that I might not be able to deliver the results they want, than to have an unhappy patient in the end. By offering an initial free consultation, our office can often refer the patient to a clinic or practice where he or she can get precisely the right care or treatment. There is a balance to be found between the doctor hearing what you want and determining that he can provide you with that kind of treatment and care. Remember, there are no guarantees in health care. In fact, there are few guarantees in life—medical or otherwise. Nevertheless, before you agree to a plan, make sure that the chiropractic doctor or your MD has the sense that he or she can help you achieve your goals.

Again, some chiropractors deal with problems that are not directly related to the spine. Maybe the patient has a condition and thinks that chiropractic care might help. Sometimes a patient just needs to see us and we will recommend a specialist.

That doesn't mean that we won't see him (or her). However, in cases where there is or could be a serious medical issue, I would ask that patient to first visit his medical doctor and if it's nothing serious, I would happily invite him back so we can look at our treatment options.

Our patients don't usually spend years in medical school like we do. Sometimes there are red-flag symptoms signaling a more serious problem than the patient imagined. Over years of cases, some patients have called me later to say thanks for sending them elsewhere, because the problem was something that needed to be checked by a specialist and would not have been successfully addressed in their chiropractic care. A physician's responsibility is to think of the patients first. By referring them to the provider who should check them first, the mystery issue should be cleared up. When they're cleared to move forward with chiropractic care, they can come back and get the treatments that they initially sought. If the issue happens to be something unrelated to chiropractic care, we want to let them know. In the end, they're happier patients. Even if you didn't actually treat them, it still builds your credibility.

SOME BENEFITS OF CHIROPRACTIC CARE

Once we've evaluated the patient and have determined that they are a candidate for chiropractic care, we present some of its many potential benefits.

Pain is one of the common reasons that a patient visits a chiropractor. Depending on the part of the body that hurts, our first job is to do a proper examination and consultation, which usually involves taking x-rays. The film helps us to rule out any other pathologies and gives us an illustration of the patient's types of spinal conditions from a bony or musculoskeletal view. The treatment stems from this process.

The benefits of treatment can be remarkable for patients who have presented conditions that couldn't be satisfactorily addressed with more "traditional medical care". Chiropractic care has been very successful in treating pain that stems from headaches, neck pain, arm pain, numbness, tingling, traditional back pain, shoulder, and knee pain—to name a few. Therefore, getting chiropractic care in conjunction with physical therapy modalities and rehabilitative techniques can add value to basic chiropractic care. If we can't relieve the pain 100%, we can usually offer pain relief, such as reducing chronic types of long-term pain or decreasing the pain to a more tolerable or more controlled level. That's very rewarding.

The benefits of chiropractic care go so much further than just pain control, especially for chronic and/or acute pain. We can also treat recent soft tissue injuries relating to areas such as the neck, the shoulders, or the knees. Chiropractic and physical therapy can be used to help strengthen the tissues and muscles and strengthen core muscle groups for a better recovery, especially for old injuries. Any time that you have a traumatic injury to tissue, there's the potential and possibility for a combination of things to happen.

For example, scar-tissue can form around an old injury, creating "adhesions", which can restrict your range of motion over time. Keeping old joint injuries supple and mobile is part of any wellness plan. Wellness care can mean anything from maintaining the spine to keeping a chronic problem at bay.

Chiropractic care can help over the long term when we proactively work to ensure that the patient continues to maintain range of motion and continuing rehydration of the discs. This is particularly important in a patient who has a degenerative condition as well as those who are feeling the effects of age. By combining chiropractic and physical therapy modalities, we've been able to slow down that degenerative process. We are actually creating changes in the disc through rehydration.

Think of the discs in your spine as little sponges that require a certain amount of fluid. That fluid level maintains itself for years but begins to drop off when you reach 52 to 55 years of age. A disc is made up of 80% water; and as we age, it dries out, depositing less fluid into the disc. Each person has 24 of those discs or "sponges" in the spine. Over time, as part of the natural aging process, they actually grow thinner—making you physically shorter.

To understand degeneration of the discs better, consider this. If you left a wet sponge on a window sill and went on vacation for a month, you'd come back and it would be pretty dried out. However, you could stick it under the faucet to get it wet and it would become soft and spongy again. If you left that same sponge on the window-sill for maybe three or four months, that sponge would dry out to the point where it would become too hard to salvage. It would just crumble. Our discs are similar. In the first half of our lives, they have an ample supply of fluids and necessary oxygen. This keeps the disc spongy and healthy. Once that dehydration begins, you experience more wear and tear. One of the benefits of chiropractic care is continuing hydration to the discs and the spine.

Some of our patients do see the benefits of "maintenance chiropractic care". Although we only see these folks once a month or so, that's enough treatment to keep hydration flowing through those discs, the spine, and the joints; so there's a better range of motion throughout their spine. Through ongoing chiropractic care of the spine, utilizing manipulative techniques plus therapeutic modalities and traction on the spine, we're actually able to increase ranges of motion to the joints of the spine, which leaves the body in a healthier long-term state.

We like to see both kinds of patients: those who want the long-term benefit of chiropractic maintenance care and those in pain who really only want acute care. For them, we attempt to relieve the pain, fix them, and put them back together. We usually don't see these patients until they return in more pain.

WHO IS THE CHIROPRACTIC PATIENT?

Demographically, our patients are a mixed bag. Even though I practice in Florida and people assume that my practice is Medicare-based and focused on the elderly, most of my patients fall within the 30- to 55-year age range. Of course, we also see younger and older patients, but most of them fall somewhere in the middle.

We do very well treating pediatric cases, depending upon the condition. In teenagers, scoliosis is a common problem. Chiropractic benefits are great for patients with a curvature on the spine. When we catch them early enough—10 to 12 years old—we have had an excellent success rate in many cases. With young people between 12 and 18 years old, we also treat many typical sports injuries.

There does come a point when our ability to help a patient is diminished, which has to do with age and previous care and lifestyle. We have a fairly small percentage of the 65- to 80-year-old group. Many of them find big benefits in chiropractic care. Unfortunately, some of them have waited too long and permanent damage is already done. There's only so much we can do for them. If older patients are looking for some pain relief and some preventive care, we can provide those services. However, sometimes their problems are so chronic and their expectations are far too high to be reachable goals because they have simply waited too long.

My preference definitely centers on treating the 30- to 55-year-olds, and they make up a majority of our practice. The body's ability to heal is so much better at an earlier age, and these patients are more physically active. Also, this age group can reap the benefits of long-term care, so we stand an excellent chance of giving them a better long-term quality of life. Statistically, these folks will need help with work-related injuries, falls, injuries such as sprains and strains, and car accidents.

This group also includes the typical, sitting-too-long-at-the-office group who go home to transform into "weekend warriors". They do yard work, like mowing the lawn and cutting the trees, or something very physical, like hiking or biking. Since they haven't done anything physical in a while, they end up spraining, straining, and hurting themselves. These people can enjoy big benefits from chiropractic care. If we can get them started earlier on the benefits of long-term chiropractic care as a wellness plan, their lives will be better overall.

TRAUMATIC TYPE INJURIES

We treat many people who have been injured in accidents, including automobile accidents, as long as there are no fractures, dislocations, or head injuries. These can be ruled out immediately through the proper diagnostic work-up including consultation, examination, and x-rays. After we've cleared our patients and are certain that there are no neurological problems, we can implement chiropractic care and physical therapy modalities.

Chiropractic is one of the best treatments for a typical car accident. We see a lot of whiplash injuries, which happen when the weight of the head (between 10 and 20 pounds) gets tossed around on the very small, soft tissue structure of the neck. Current laws require us to be locked in with seatbelts and shoulder harnesses. Some of our patients wonder if the safety gear contributes to their injury. This may happen on rare occasions, but most of the time it saves lives. There are far more stories about saved lives from the use of seat belts, shoulder harnesses, air bags, and similar equipment.

After 35 years of experience, I have a historical perspective on this particular problem. Years ago, patients who were in accidents came to us after their release from the hospital, where they had been treated for head injuries from contact with windshields, chest contusions, punctured lungs, etc. Life-threatening injuries have been reduced dramatically by using seat belts, shoulder harnesses, and air bags. There are also far fewer severe neurological injuries. From our perspective, today's accident victims are much better off because they tend to suffer only from soft tissue injuries.

Musculoskeletal injuries or soft tissue injuries (whiplash, pinched nerves, and disc injuries) are a lot less devastating and easier to treat than neurological head trauma. Seat belts and shoulder harnesses lock the body into place, but we still haven't figured out how to strap the head in completely and still allow them to drive and see. So after a 30-mile-per-hour hit from the rear, your body locks up, the seat belt locks up, but your 10- to 20-pound head still bounces back and forth like a bowling ball on your neck. This leads to tearing and stretching of the neck's soft tissue, which creates injury to the ligaments causing a weakness that we call whiplash. In these accidents, the normal cervical curve gets flattened or reversed. Then the rest of the spine is securely locked into place but will still absorb the impact and some compression which can cause potential injury to the lower spine.

Some studies show that the accidents causing spinal compression can create some nerve irritation that moves through the spine, the neck, down the mid-back to the lower back and beyond. Another condition we see in car accidents are the result of the patient's hands bracing on the steering wheel at the time of the accident. Some shoulder impingement occurs when the shoulder socket gets jammed from the force of locking in place while your hands keep a death-grip on the steering wheel. These are some of the musculoskeletal injuries that occur as a result of typical auto accidents.

Chiropractic care specializes in those kinds of soft tissue injuries. Soft tissue injury is probably what we do best. We can work wonders by bringing in physical therapy, manipulation adjustments, traction, and decompression. This is especially true for patients who have been experiencing pinched nerves, tingling, radiating pain, headaches, or numbness.

Even in more serious cases, when we do MRIs and find bulging herniated discs, we can continue to treat our patients unless the condition shows severe neurological symptoms such as a loss of bladder or bowel control or foot drop. Nevertheless, most chiropractors doing a proper evaluation can discern those kinds of issues. We can treat those patients with bulging herniated discs, whether we use our spinal decompression machine or cervical traction (for cervical and lumbar types of disc injury). If we get to the point of feeling that we can do no more, that patient might be a candidate for Epidural Steroid Injection. If that injection isn't successful, the patient might be a candidate for some form of decompression surgery.

We've had great results with our spinal decompression machine. Even patients who were scheduled for surgical consultations, after hearing about other patients' success in using the machine, have wanted to try this less invasive technique. That's been a real benefit to our patients and our practice.

So when it comes to accident injuries, chiropractic is probably the first line of defense I would recommend. In soft tissue damage, we can get our patients to a place where they feel a good deal of fast relief. We also work closely with a medical doctor who comes in and does trigger point injections and medications when necessary. We utilize all of the tools at our disposal to make sure that the patient gets the best benefits of care.

TECHNOLOGICALLY SPEAKING

Technology is improving our ability to treat our patients effectively, and over the years we have had some tried and true techniques to help our patients. One such was "manipulation under anesthesia". We did this on patients with severe conditions who haven't responded to other forms of therapy and chiropractic manipulation. When we cannot help the patient because of the pain they feel, or because they cannot relax for fear that they *might* be hurt, we work with an outpatient surgery center to administer the necessary twilight anesthesia prior to the manipulation. The medical profession has long used this technique as a treatment for frozen shoulders and other joints.

I was been certified to do this years ago This technique allows us to get a lot more range of motion and work on patients with very painful conditions such as fibromyalgia and disc injuries. We also use it on patients with severe and chronic back problems, like severe scar-tissue adhesions and for some who had failed back surgery. This successful technique can be used for certain conditions by bringing the patient's spine through a painless range of motion that could not normally be reached while the patient was awake.

Today, chiropractors are also increasing their use of laser therapy. In our office, we use laser therapy under certain conditions where the technology helps to speed up the healing of tissue. Around 12 to 15 years ago, we were among the first in Palm Beach County to begin using the spinal decompression machine when it first came out. Now, a few different machines can be used to do spinal de-compressive therapy. This upgraded form of traction can decompress spinal components without involving the the pulling of the muscles.

You may be wondering how long these treatments take. Spinal decompression begins with an average number of sessions— typically between 20 and 24 visits at about three times per week. Of course, this depends upon the patient's symptoms, and the severity of the condition. However, after utilizing the decompression for as long as we have, we now do a halfway evaluation: after 12 visits, we begin to look for beneficial signs before we commit the patient to further treatment.

With time, and after using certain techniques, we get a better understanding of expected timelines. Procedures like manipulation under anesthesia will take only three days. I have had patients who return three or four years later, saying they are still doing well from the procedure. This process has given us excellent benefits and given the patient long-term relief without the need to return.

A good doctor will look at the patient's condition and see the patient as an individual. That doctor will look at findings from previous exams and current x-rays, and after looking at the history, will find the treatment plan that fits the needs of that individual. I've never viewed any particular treatment as a one type, one-stop shop for everybody. I believe treatment needs to be individualized based upon a patient's history and condition.

So, again, one can see that it is very important for patients to have access to a chiropractor who is on top of the available technology. In terms of using new technology, we test it first: if it helps us reach our patients' goals, then we will utilize it. If it doesn't, then we won't. Our goal will always be to achieve the best possible benefit for our patients, whatever it takes.

WHAT BRINGS PATIENTS TO CHIROPRACTORS?

Musculoskeletal complaints come in all forms like muscle spasm of the neck or strain of the muscle. Typically, those are the simpler conditions. If it's a new pain, it could be just a simple sprain or strain caused by some activity. We will do a thorough evaluation and examination, and then we take x-rays of the area to see what's going on. The patient starts treatment quickly and usually the benefits are quickly evident with these kinds of complaints, the patient can be in and out of the office within a couple of days to weeks.

Joint injuries are usually ligamentous tears and are worse than just a sprain, meaning there will be more care and treatment involved in joint-related complaints. With the mid- to low-back area, a musculoskeletal spasm could be just an acute symptom caused by sleeping or sitting too long, or just a quick muscle spasm. In theory, after an evaluation and a few visits, we can get the patient in and out of the process without sustaining any chronic or long-term issues.

OTHER CHIROPRACTIC CANDIDATES

There are many different conditions that chiropractors can treat after conducting a good evaluation. Sometimes our patient displays something musculoskeletal along with potential neurological issues. For example, patients sometimes arrive with symptoms like headaches for which chiropractic care works wonders, but they are also complaining of ringing in the ears, dizziness, and maybe even vertigo. This may be related to a separate condition and perhaps they have heard that chiropractors can help with this. I would first make sure that the patient has already visited with an Ear Nose and Throat (ENT) specialist, and that he has ruled out any internal ear damage. If the dizziness and vertigo relates to a non-neurological condition, it could be something that's occurring inside the ear that we could help with chiropractic care.

There are tiny calcium crystals that look like tiny grains of sand which are in your inner ear. These can also create some "positional" vertigo and dizziness when they have been disrupted, which can be disconcerting to the patient. The patient might be standing up or lying down and suddenly become dizzy and nauseous. Once we've ruled out that the condition is not a severe ENT medical issue, I have treated many of those cases with great success. Basically, we put their head through some range of motion and shift those little crystals back to where they belong in the inner ear, and the complaint goes away.

Other ear problems respond well to chiropractic care. Often, when children get chronic ear infections in their early years, doctors suggest having tubes put into the ears. Sometimes we can avoid this invasive surgery by using manipulative therapy to the cervical spine. There is a direct relationship between the nervous system and the neck to the inner ear. I make sure that the parent has first taken the child to a pediatrician and that the MD has ruled out any other conditions. Then I can treat the child.

Over the years, I have treated numerous medical conditions. I prefer to err on the side of caution and always rule out any serious medical condition at first. Once those have been ruled out, I have no problems using chiropractic care to treat not just musculoskeletal conditions but also some other medical conditions that historically benefit from chiropractic care: stomach issues, constipation, menstrual cycles, and other female reproductive problems.

Chiropractors often get referrals from OB/GYNs when the mother is having back pain, neck pain, or headaches. She can't take medication while she's pregnant, but we can still adjust her spine. We can still do certain types of treatment on her: manual traction, muscular trigger point work, and massage, etc. We can offer the benefits of some pain relief until the day she gives birth; chiropractic care even does well for labor pain.

Again with other medical issues, after very cautiously ruling out any of the more serious medical conditions, our office has treated everything from constipation to abdominal pain, we can also treat with success children who have been diagnosed with ADHD and hyperactive syndrome. We do this for those parents who adamantly don't want their children on some of the available medications. The adjustments have a calming effect on the child's spine and the entire nervous system.

Chiropractic treatment for the nervous system to create a calming effect really expresses the whole premise of chiropractic care, which is all about helping the nervous system to function properly throughout the spine. We can make sure that there is a flow of communication going from all of the parts of the body to the other parts of the body. When there is an uninterrupted flow of nerve impulses, that's when healing happens. Chiropractic has a major effect on the nervous system which ultimately affects everything in the body. The disruption or injury creates the interference in the nervous system, and that's where we focus our attention with our chiropractic adjustments and treatment.

WHAT EXACTLY IS AN ADJUSTMENT?

Sometimes chiropractors will call what we do by way of manipulation to the spine an "adjustment". It can be done in a number of different ways. Chiropractors have a lot of different techniques to manipulate the spine. Most chiropractors are fairly well-versed in all of the techniques. For example, I have either taken courses or learned most of the latest trends and techniques over the last 35 years. This way, if somebody comes in with special needs, we can help him or her.

An adjustment is the manipulative aspect of chiropractic care and the result of applied pressure—a force through the spinal joint in the body that corresponds to a specific level of the spine where the problem lies. This manipulation opens up, makes limber, and separates tissue around the spine, increasing the blood and oxygen flow as well as the nerve supply to that area. There are forceful techniques and non-force techniques, some of which involve chiropractic tools that can adjust the spine. The chiropractor chooses the technique to fit the adjustment to the patient. Some patients are comfortable with a more forceful technique and others are not.

In "lumbar rolls"—cervical adjustments—we manually move things around using the back of our hands. Some people call it "popping" because sometimes there is an audible sound as the pressure is released in the joint area. People sometimes get alarmed by that noise. They'll say something like, "What was that popping?" or, "I don't want my neck cracked." Most chiropractors don't care for the term "cracked". It sounds violent. The sound is just what happens when something that's been stuck in an uncomfortable position becomes un-stuck.

Depending upon whether the patient is a 10-year-old boy with very small joints or an 80-year-old with osteoporosis, chiropractors fit the adjustment to the patient. Non-forceful adjustments on the spinal joints can also achieve the necessary change that affects the nervous system and ultimately changes the symptoms. We also have various tables that we use for different purposes such as drop tables and stretching tables. The chiropractor has a good sized tool-box that can be used to make that adjustment a good experience.

CAN EXERCISE MAKE A DIFFERENCE?

Exercise can make your body healthier in many ways. I always give my patients an exercise program to do at home as they are able, to reintegrate exercise into their lives—from lower back stretch techniques to chest stretches. People in this country are plagued with back problems. I'm convinced that if people were to do some of the basic daily or twice-daily exercises that we show them, on the floor or on the bed, it would alleviate a lot of future problems. Back problems happen because of the tightening and shortening of our muscles. In the past two hundred years, we've become a very sedentary population. We drive everywhere, we don't ride bicycles, and this lack of motion makes our muscles shrink and tighten up—especially if we don't stretch.

Europeans are quite different. Elderly people over there are in a lot better shape than our older folks. They don't sit on their bums behind a desk all day, which has a profound effect on the musculoskeletal system. Europeans walk up and down hills to go shopping and either walk or ride bicycles to get around.

Think of your body as a spring that is winding tighter and tighter, year after year. As our muscles get tighter and shorter, we're actually creating more compression on our spines. Compression on our spines will create wear and tear. That's where we get the onset of degenerative arthritis. In the animal kingdom, you'll notice that most animals don't develop arthritis. No, they don't ride bicycles, but they do move around. Since they are on all fours, gravity is pushing down on their spine and actually helping to keep open their spine and joints because of the way they walk on four legs.

Since humans stand on two legs, the force of gravity is pushing directly down on our heads to our spine for our entire lives. What happens with that pressure? It compresses our spine and the discs in between. Let's add up all of those factors. We have a shortening and compression effect on our spine, we're sitting all day and not moving our joints, and our bodies have begun to tighten and wear out faster. When you eventually go to a chiropractor, he gives you exercises. He can explain and show you how to stretch, bend out, roll the spine, and then open up various muscles (iliolumbar and piriformis) and the lateral portion of the lower legs.

Exercise is terribly important. Chiropractors can give their patients any number of basic exercises that could act as steps to wellness if they would just do a few twice a day. I've been using them most of my life. I've not had many spinal problems. I believe that it is the combination of getting regular chiropractic care maintenance and exercising that keeps me going.

UNDERSTANDING CHIROPRACTIC STANDARDS

Sometimes patients are not convinced that chiropractors have been educated to the same degree as their medical peers. When we are in school, we all cover the same material. If you took the time to compare the curriculum, you would see that chiropractors go to the same classes that are required in medical schools. The only real difference is that we spend a lot more time on the musculoskeletal system and anatomy while our medical brothers and sisters spend their time learning about drugs and pharmacology.

Since we do not prescribe medication, we don't have to spend time on learning about the positives and negatives of medications, the drugs themselves, and their possible interactions. We spend more of our time on the musculoskeletal aspect of the spine and the nervous system, which makes us more proficient than a traditional medical doctor when talking about the spine or musculoskeletal systems.

People don't necessarily know this, but it's definitely important to understand. All of the basic courses in medical school are required; we actually log more hours, do an internship, and must be licensed in each state where we practice—just like other doctors. We also must take and pass national board and state board exams. Every few years, chiropractors also have to do a CA accreditation to maintain an active license. That just gives people the basic under-standing that a chiropractor has the education and requirements up to an acceptable medical standard.

HOW LONG DO YOU HAVE TO TREAT WITH A CHIROPRACTOR?

From time to time we hear people say, "If you go to a chiropractor, you have to go for the rest of your life." Chiropractic care can be a lifelong benefit but it's not required. That's always up to the patient. Chiropractors, myself included, hope to educate our patients about what can or cannot be done through chiropractic care and the benefits they can look forward to. Understanding chiropractic care can allow a patient to help the patient choose the best form of treatment for his or her specific condition.

Over the years, I have seen patients' care moving in the direction of wellness, particularly when they've had repetitive conditions or injuries, or see the same conditions come back again. It's like a learning experience. We tell them, "This is what's going on; if you do this, it will keep you going." Sometimes, it takes a patient a longer period of time to discover and thoroughly understand that there are long-term benefits created by long-term chiropractic care.

After practicing for 35 years, it's easy for me to say this emphatically because I've had patients who have been coming to me for treatment from my first years in practice. These folks have seen and felt the benefits of chiropractic. Without question, they're in better physical shape than their peers who haven't had the benefits of years of chiropractic care. You just can't ignore the benefits of including chiropractic care in your life.

AND FINALLY

I can only hope that this information allows potential patients to have a better understanding of Chiropractic Care and its benefits.
I also want to thank all my patients, past and present, over the last 35 years who have had the foresight to seek out chiropractic care and who have given me the pleasure of treating them.

(This content should be used for informational purposes only. It does not create a doctor-patient relationship with any reader and should not be construed as medical advice. If you need medical advice, please contact a doctor in your community who can assess the specifics of your situation.)

9

THE WHOLE YOU – APPRECIATING YOUR OWN COMPLEXITIES

by Christopher J. Bump, D.C.

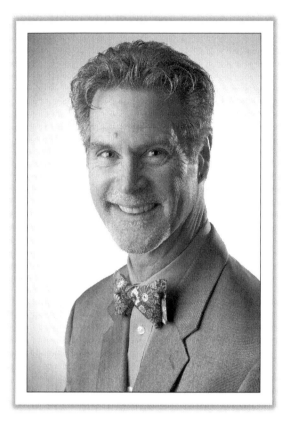

Christopher J. Bump, D.C.
Christopher J. Bump, D.C.
Mcafee, New Jersey
www.drbump.com

Dr. Christopher Bump graduated at the top of his class from Palmer College in 1982, earning the distinct honor of being the Clinic Intern Director overseeing other doctors in the school's health clinic. More recently, Dr. Bump earned a Master's Degree in human nutrition from Columbia University. Having studied nutritional biochemistry and clinical nutrition, he can see the interaction of all the organs, glands, tissues and systems of the body, which is critical when diagnosing and treating patients.

Dr. Bump is first and foremost a healer of the whole individual, offering a truly holistic approach to medicine. He is concerned with not only eliminating symptoms, but also creating a total health and well-being plan for his patients.

THE WHOLE YOU – APPRECIATING YOUR OWN COMPLEXITIES

I grew up in the 1950s and 60s when our country was going through a sort of identity crisis, much like a teen does. The status quo was being questioned on many different levels, including the Vietnam War, civil rights, women's rights, and health care. Because I was a teen in the tumultuous 1960s, it is not surprising to me that I learned to question the status quo, especially established industrial complexes such as medicine, pharmaceuticals, and agriculture. As a result, my educational path and interests led me down some very interesting roads, one of which was the concept of "Alternative Medicine." So in my late teens and early 20s, I began an exploration of organic foods and herbal therapy, which led me to the work of some early pioneers in the field that became my influence: Linus Pauling, Carlton Fredericks, Bernarr Macfadden, Herbert Shelton, Adelle Davis, etc.

Early in my adult life, I became disenchanted with traditional medicine. It seemed to me then—and it is worse today—that most medical professionals, as well intended as they may be, view patients only as a collection of symptoms to be treated.

There is no interest, or perhaps ability, in investigating the underlying causes of a patient's condition. To me, even as a young, inquisitive student, knowing how a patient developed their condition would be the key to healing it. As an example, my chronic sinus congestion did not clear up until I eliminated the cause, which, for me, was dairy. Regardless of all the sprays and herbal tinctures I took, it was not until I stopped consuming casein, which is one of the main proteins in dairy food, that I found relief. Casein is the primary protein used in the manufacturing of glues. This is why Elsie's picture is on the front of Elmer's glue! So, from the very beginning of my interest in medicine, that deeper search to discover the cause was important to me.

In my 20s, I was introduced to chiropractic care through a friend who had gastro-intestinal problems. She suffered from bleeding ulcers and was being treated by a chiropractor who used nutritional therapies in his practice. This really piqued my interest, as I had never seen an actual "doctor" who took a more natural, non-medical approach to healing his patients. I asked to come along to one of her office visits, and I was exposed to an entirely new world of health care delivery. Her appointment was focused primarily on diet and remedies she could do at home to help her. She did have a chiropractic adjustment, which was also new to me, but most of her appointment was discussing lifestyle changes. Meditation was also recommended because it, he further explained, "helped to reduce stress, and ulcers were a result of the stress response." I have never forgotten that comment as it changed my life forever, as it opened up an entirely new understanding for me about cause and effect. Remember, this was the early 70s! He also prescribed remedies I considered a bit peculiar but that I later learned were based on the work of Edgar Cayce—an early 20th-century healer who enjoyed an amazing career in bringing wellness to people in non-traditional ways.

Edgar Cayce was a fascinating man, raised in a traditional Southern Baptist environment, but he possessed a gift that was beyond our understanding. Some would call him a psychic, others a medium, but, to me, he simply channeled the graces of God. He recommended all-natural remedies, including both osteopathic and chiropractic adjustments. Having little understanding of either approach, I began an exploration of both professions and discovered that osteopathy had changed its philosophical and ideological principles to ones of a more medical approach. Chiropractic, on the other hand, acknowledged the concept of innate intelligence while encouraging a hands-on approach to healing, and this really appealed to me.

My initial exposure to this alternative approach to health care opened my eyes, mind, and soul to my life-long prayer: to be of service to others. I graduated from Palmer College in 1982, where I continued to study nutrition and soft-tissue techniques. Even then I questioned the traditional chiropractic concepts of "subluxation" and "nerve root impingement," as scientifically they did not make sense. However, understanding how the muscle, connective tissue, ligaments, and tendons influenced joint mobility and function made perfect sense to me. I am surprised I made it through chiropractic college, as I was always questioning the traditional explanation of how chiropractic works. I'd simply ask, "What causes a subluxation?" Even then, over 30 years ago, I also knew that a person's life choices and events would affect everything about their health, whether it was eating refined white bread and lots of sugar, overusing their upper body with weight training, or worrying about their children or social issues. What we do, think, feel, and believe has everything to do with the balance of our health.

So, even in the early days of study and career, I was passionately certain that diet, lifestyle, and nutrition mattered in the overall health of my patients. Eventually, I developed what I call a holographic model for working with patients, because it acknowledges the complete uniqueness of each and every patient and addresses not only their physical health but also their spiritual and emotional health. My education continues even today, including a master's degree in nutrition from Columbia University and a fellowship in acupuncture. More recently, I've become a certified functional medical practitioner through the Institute of Functional Medicine. This eclectic and holistic approach to health care has created for me (and hopefully my patients) a very comprehensive and systematic way of helping my patients find better health.

TREATING THE WHOLE PATIENT

The difference in how I approach each patient begins immediately when we consult for the first time. Since my concern is for the whole person, my primary interest is to get to know my patient. I need to know their story, what life events caused them to be sitting in my office with their plethora of health concerns. It may be chronic ear infections or strep throat from childhood leading to overuse of antibiotics, having mono in high school, or poor eating habits throughout their lifetime. My initial interview with a patient involves one to two hours of sitting down and learning about her (or his) life in general. We discuss their primary concerns, but also I want to learn how they have traveled along life's path. I need to understand the sources of stress, toxicity, fatigue, hormonal imbalance, etc., not just the headache or neck pain. I need to know what her everyday life looks like; how she eats, and what she does for recreation and relaxation.

My medical colleagues attempt to describe conditions or symptoms as a "disease." In traditional allopathic medicine, they give the symptoms a name and then call that a disease and blame the disease for causing the symptoms. Arthritis is an example. A patient comes into the doctor's office complaining of joint pain in the neck, low back or shoulder. The doctor tells them they have arthritis, which they do, because arthritis is literally "inflammation of a joint." The symptoms are named, and this becomes the disease. The patient asks, "What causes this?" and the reply is, "Arthritis causes the inflammation and pain, and you have arthritis." The patient then asks, "What can I do about this?" and the reply is, "Take an anti-inflammatory medicine or get an adjustment, as this will stop the pain and inflammation." However, in truth, the remedy only treats the symptoms, which, in this case, is an inflammation of the joint. In the typical allopathic model, only the symptoms are addressed. This is true not only medically, but also in the chiropractic profession. A spinal or joint adjustment to reduce pain is not any different than taking an aspirin. I prefer to think in terms of imbalance. Patients become unwell because they've been pushed out of balance. This approach can apply to any aspect of their being: emotional, mental, structural, or even spiritual. It is necessary to look beyond the symptoms to the patient as a whole who has walked through life. A person with a history and circumstances, choices, and decisions that have ultimately created an imbalance expressed in all the signs and symptoms which brought them into my office: muscle tension, digestive disorder, hormonal imbalance, etc. In my example above with arthritis, we look at all the possible reasons the joint is inflamed.

This may include an overuse pattern from stress at work, or toxins from a microbe like Lyme or Epstein–Barr virus, or it could be from dehydration or a nutrient deficiency such as magnesium or essential fatty acids.

Stress is a greater cause of our modern health problems, but not just the obvious, like life-threatening events. Nutritional excess and deficiency are stressors, as is driving down the highway at 70 mph. Worrying about our children or world events and not getting proper rest are stressors as well. Our bodies have a predictable response to stress. When we are threatened or *think* we may be threatened, the body goes into the "fight or flight" response. Almost instantly, our system receives an increased stimulation of adrenaline that enables us to either run away as fast as we can or to stay and fight with the source of the stress. Even though there are no more saber-toothed tigers to battle with, our body's response to stress still uses the same physical, neurological, and endocrine response pathways. Our bodies don't differentiate between good stress and bad stress. Your body reacts to the positive stress of getting married in two hours in exactly the same way as if you have your life threatened in a dark alleyway. There is a powerful hormonal (adrenaline) and neurologic response to stress, and all our energy and our blood supply is rerouted to our legs and arms so that we can run or fight to save ourselves. The stress response diverts our normal, healthy functioning to a survival mode, so most of our normal organ and hormonal functions become skewed in fear for our survival. What I mean is we don't need to digest food when we are running for our lives, nor is it sensible to be considering making love to our partner when we are running for our lives. You get the picture. Our body goes into survival mode and the luxury systems are put on hold. Even the thyroid gland responds to chronic stress by shutting down. Stress, when it lingers day after day, can be seriously damaging to all of our systems.

As scientists and researchers study the killer conditions of our day, stress seems to be an important causal link. Stress has been linked to cancer, diabetes, heart disease, obesity, and even musculoskeletal issues. Stress certainly plays a part in automobile accidents and cardiac events. As chiropractors begin to understand how overall health can be affected by stress or other chemistry-modifying circumstances, we get closer to treating the patient at a much more elemental level. The patient may be presented with structural symptoms like headaches or back pain, but that pain may be related to an emotional, mental, or spiritual imbalance that is expressing itself structurally.

I know it sounds "New Agey," but we are all interrelated through a matrix that really connects us to the entire universe. Actually, we know this scientifically. Max Planck, who was a friend and colleague of Albert Einstein's, explains it this way. He said in 1944,

> *"All matter originates and exists only by virtue of a force, which brings the particle of an atom to vibration and holds this most minute solar system of the atom together. We must assume behind this force the existence of a conscious and intelligent mind. This mind is the matrix of all matter."*

I mention this because there is so much that influences our health, and it is up to us to both understand and use that which we know to help us maintain balanced health. Changing how and what we eat is important, but so is what we feel and what we believe. Prayer, meditation, love, and compassion must be an integral part of everyone's healing path.

TECHNICALLY SPEAKING

I want to tell you the story of one of my patients, but first I need to share a few concepts. It is important that we understand that cells communicate with each other in several important ways.

Chiropractic care begins with the understanding that a person is a compilation of trillions of cells that are supposed to work in a synergistic, harmonious way; our organs and glands are not isolated components. Also, the body has "innate intelligence" etched within our DNA—an ability to self-regulate, self-heal, and maintain. (This is not just a chiropractic principle.) Sometimes our wounds need to be stitched up, but we don't really have to manipulate the healing process. Structure and function are intimately related, so the structure of our body dictates function and vice versa.

For example, every one of the 100 trillion cells in our body has a cellular membrane. The structure of that membrane is integral to its function. There are protein receptors that are essential for cellular communication, for instance, that sit within the cell wall. If the cell wall of a membrane is unable to hold these receptor proteins, then cell signaling suffers. The structural architecture of the cell membrane is totally dependent on proper levels of essential fatty acids and also cholesterol. We're taught that cholesterol is a bad and dangerous molecule that should be eliminated. But, as mentioned above, cholesterol is an essential component of the structural integrity of our cellular membrane. So, structure affects function.

Also, function affects structure, for example if your muscles and connective tissue are exceedingly tight and contracted. Because muscles both move and stabilize joints, they will affect the body's structure. If a muscle is always tight pulling through a joint, it will, over time, begin to affect how the joint moves. Imagine the support ropes on a circus tent cinched much tighter on one end. The tent would pull lopsided to one side and may eventually collapse. A simple example of how function will affect the structure is tight muscles affecting the movement and stability of a joint, whether it be a neck, low back, or shoulder.

When chiropractors are treating a patient who has joint misalignment or fixation, they must, in my opinion, look at all of the supportive tissues around that joint. It is not enough to try and isolate and adjust a spinal joint without evaluating why they are misaligned. Evaluating the function-structure relation is essential. Since the ligaments, tendons, muscles, and connective tissue support and move joints, these components of structural integrity must be evaluated. Every element is intimately related. Unless we address the soft tissue along with the joint, we do the patient a disservice. Imbalances affect function in any tissue, gland, or cell. This understanding of structure and function works from not only the gross anatomical level, but also right down to the inner organelle of the cells, so that the concept of imbalance can be applied throughout the entire body—from the joints right down to the nuclear DNA.

It's pretty easy to understand that an injury, trauma, or overuse (like working out too hard in the gym) may lead to a soft tissue injury. It's more difficult to associate emotional, mental, or even spiritual stresses with a chain of imbalances. Worrying is an example of a chronic stress, as is commuting, being fearful of a crazed religious group, working 12 hour days, or fearing death or aging. Remember, regardless of the source of stress, our body always responds as if it is the saber-toothed tiger. Stress response leads to increased muscular tightness and inflammation, which in turn leads to dysfunction in our joints, which can develop aches and pains. I hope this explanation helps explain that many of the causes of their aches, tensions, and types of fatigue are non-physical.

More specifically, if someone is emotionally distraught and going through a stress response as a result of a relationship issue with a spouse, the body's fight or flight response will kick in. That initial stress response is caused by adrenaline and the stimulation of part of the nervous system called the "sympathetic nervous system," which creates muscle tightness and readiness for either fleeing or fighting. If you extend that intense condition of continual low-grade stress over a period of weeks or months, something has to give. Often, it's the occipital bone in the back of the head (causing tension headache) or tightened muscles in the upper back and neck (cervical spine restriction), leading to the need for chiropractic care.

If you're still with me, let's get specific.

BARBARA

I had a patient whose name was Barbara. She was a 58-year-old retired schoolteacher who had years and years of headaches and pain in both the upper and lower back area and the neck. She had been a chiropractic patient for many years, loved the profession, and loved being adjusted. But Barbara was getting adjustments week in, week out, often two times a week! She thought that this was a very normal thing in the realm of chiropractic care. Eventually, she came into my office because she was told that I work a little differently with my patients.

In my initial interview with her, I asked her if she ever stopped to think about why she needed chiropractic adjustments so regularly. The rest of the conversation went something like this:

> "Of course, well, I go out," she answered.
> "What do you mean 'you go out'?" I asked.
> "Well, my spine goes out."
> "Why does it go out?" I asked her. Barbara
>   had no answer.

I suggested that perhaps there was some other imbalance leading to the sensation that her spine was going out. Perhaps her muscles were too tight and inflamed. Perhaps there were other health components that might be contributing to her pain, which she hadn't really looked at.

Barbara was not interested in considering that idea.

I said that I would work with her from a structural point of view, but I asked her to remain open to the possibility that there might be underlying metabolic causes for her condition and chronic pain. She agreed to that treatment approach, so I started working with her. Almost immediately, her pain levels were reduced significantly. Eventually, she only needed to come into the office for an adjustment once every two or three weeks.

Later, I reminded her of our initial conversation and suggested that it might be time to look into some metabolic causes for her pain. She agreed. After a lab work-up, we discovered that she had a very high inflammatory marker in her body. She had a low-grade rheumatoid factor elevation as well. Her thyroglob-ulin antibodies were elevated, her hemoglobin levels were high, and she also had an undiscovered autoimmune thyroid issue.

Barbara had other symptoms not necessarily tied to her pain. She had gained two pounds on average for each of the past 15 years, making her about 40 pounds overweight. She was not sleeping, allergies were a constant issue, and she suffered chronic infections. She was feeling old, but she was only a 58-year-old retired educator—her body hadn't been abused by heavy lifting or factory-type work.

I suggested that we do some lifestyle and nutritional work around the symptoms, so we started with a significant lifestyle change. We took her off of "antigenic foods"—foods frequently associated with allergies. For a month, she worked through an elimination diet and then a detoxification program, and we did a reassessment at the end of that month.

Not only were the pain and headaches gone, but also her muscles were relaxed. She lost approximately 10 pounds in the first month, and was sleeping better. She said that she felt 15 years younger, and she wanted to continue this process of lifestyle management.

Now, Barbara visits every six to eight weeks for a "de-stressing session," where I work on her muscles and connective tissues. I adjust her from time to time as needed. At this point, she has lost close to 35 pounds. She looks and feels like a different woman. This is a typical patient story. They come in with something they think is structural and find that it's a metabolic issue.

There's more to healing than meets the eye.

THE CASE FOR MECHANOTRANSDUCTION

Chiropractic care depends upon the concept of "mechanotransduction." This intimidating word merely describes the process by which cells inside their tissues sense mechanical stress and convert these stresses into biochemical signals. This relates to the prior explanation of cellular communication. Essentially, the disciplines of acupuncture and massage therapy depend upon this concept, as does chiropractic care.

One of the challenges faced by the chiropractic profession is their historic ideology and theories about how chiropractic care works. There is more than a little skepticism about the concepts of traditional chiropractic care. Nevertheless, this profession would not have survived for 120 years if it did not offer some benefit to patients. However, the concepts used by chiropractic practitioners to justify their place in medicine—such as the concept of subluxation—just don't hold up to the scrutiny of modern medical science. The antiquated subluxation concept is being debated inside and outside the discipline. In my opinion, this debate is holding the entire profession back from becoming a mainstream healing modality. Chiropractic care does have a rightful place in the world of medicine because it is the only profession that treats patients with an emphasis on wellness from a Western perspective. (Acupuncture does the same from an Eastern perspective.)

Chiropractors need to be able to point to science that defines what actually happens when someone receives a manipulation. As it happens, there is an entire science dedicated to studying the cell-to-cell signaling that occurs as a result of pressures upon the body. It's called mechanotransduction. In a broader sweep, it's also called "mechanobiology." Practitioners of acupuncture, massage therapy, and chiropractic care are performing the science of mechanotherapy.

The body communicates internally using three different systems. One is the nervous system, another uses chemicals such as hormones and cytokines, and the third system for internal signals uses pressure or actual mechanical forces. This third branch of signaling through the body has had the least amount of attention and has the smallest body of research. Nevertheless, the research over the past 15 years on mechanotransduction is proving its scientific validity. The baroreceptors in arteries provide an example of mechanically induced signaling that is well understood and studied.

I'll keep mechanotransduction as basic as possible. Every single cell in our body is surrounded by an exterior extracellular, supportive matrix, which is comprised of pro-teins that are made up of fibroblast, meaning they are the active cells in connective tissues. There are many different kinds of these fibroblasts throughout your body, depending upon their location and their function.

This extracellular matrix has the ability, through its connection to the cell membrane, to influence what happens to that cell. Through actual mechanical pressure, 100 trillion cells will be told how to move, replicate, or divide. Sometimes there may be an over-population of cells in an area. When the pressure begins to build from cells pushing against each other, they begin to get the message: "Hey, we don't need you anymore. Self-destruct." And they do. That process is called "apoptosis." Or, there may be the need for an increase in cell division, and this will occur in tissues where the cells are moving around freely, unencumbered by life, and they begin to divide!

Any pressure on the outside of a cell wall creates an immediate signaling down through the cytoskeleton inside the cell, which then communicates to the DNA. The transmembrane proteins that connect the cell to the extracellular matrix and the cytoskeleton (which is the internetwork inside the cell) are called integrin proteins. Clusters of these integrin proteins are called focal adhesions. These little connecting proteins are the major communication highways of pressure signaling for the body. Every single cell is subject to this.

If a person is lying on the table, and a chiropractor puts pressure down onto a patient's skin, connective tissue, muscle, and joints, this pressure affects the signaling in the soft tissue and its connected joint. Therefore, if a chiropractor is manipulating the soft tissue and joints of an individual, technically it is a mechanobiological process.

I was first exposed to the science of mechanotransduction by the past president of National University, Dr. James Winterstein. Professionally, I could never understand or agree with the concepts of subluxation and nerve root impingement, which are the traditional tenets of chiropractic care. We know that chiropractic would not have survived 120 years if it did not work, and we know patients benefit from manipulation. Although I'd always known that the profession was amazing and did so much good, I'd never been able to explain how it worked until I came upon this branch of science. Without going into anything more specific, mechanobiology and mechanotransduction offer a very credible and scientific explanation for the reason chiropractic treatments affect our health.

MARYANNE

This second case is an example of a patient who visited me with more organic, non-structural concerns and conditions who also benefitted from structural manipulation.

Maryanne was a 46-year-old woman who was referred to me by a local practitioner for chronic fatigue conditions. She had been diagnosed with fibromyalgia. For 13 years, Maryanne had absolutely no energy and had lived in a constant state of aches and pains. The medic who referred her to me hoped that I could discover the causation of the fibromyalgia from an organic and glandular perspective. We discovered that she had a chronic viral overload, and a chronic microbial overload. Her adrenal glands were exhausted, her thyroid gland was not working well, and so on. She demonstrated a whole host of organic imbalances.

In addition, her muscles and connective tissues were extremely inflamed and tight. No matter where I touched Maryanne during the examination process, she experienced extreme pain. We did a work-up using a functional medicine approach and began therapies for her imbalances. I also suggested that she come in for myofascial treatments and adjustments. Chiropractic care was new to Maryanne, as she was a pharmacist by training. She had never had any kind of chiropractic work done though she had done well with an occasional massage.

Over time, I explained trigger points and the inflamed state of her muscles. I assured her that she would feel better once those trigger points were treated. I further explained that we needed to break up the tightness and tension in the muscle-connective tissue complex for her to experience any relief.

Since Maryanne lived at least an hour away, she could not see me but once every 7 to 10 days, which was not as frequent as is recommended. As mentioned above, she received myofascial therapies to break up the trigger points, adhesions, and restrictions. (These are hands-on treatments applying pressure to affected areas.) The speed of her response and her improvement in joint mobility was remarkable. Her pain quickly dissipated and her energy improved.

In functional medicine, there is an acknowledged interrelation between all the systems of the body, which includes not only structural integrity but also our emotions, thinking, and beliefs (think spiritual). We took a functional medicine approach with Maryanne, as I do with every patient. There is a matrix that exists where organ and glandular systems (such as immunity, cellular restoration, and detoxification) integrate with the structural integrity of the patient. This matrix suggests that structural integrity is an essential component of a patient's overall wellness and balance. Working with a patient like Maryanne from a structural perspective helped her to find a more efficient and quicker response to the therapies we used to balance her organ and glandular issues.

THE FUTURE OF CHIROPRACTIC CARE

As I mentioned earlier, there is ongoing chiropractic debate about how our discipline fits into the bigger health care picture. Chiropractors could easily become acknowledged and accepted as a profession if they were willing to make some ideological changes. In order for the chiropractic profession to earn its rightful place in the health delivery arena, and to stop being viewed as second-rate health care providers, the profession as a whole needs to do some adjusting of their own.

Since the Affordable Care Act, millions of people without access to health care can now be treated. In the future, the need for primary care doctors will mushroom alongside a major shortage. This is due in part because most young doctors finishing residency are interested in specialization, where they can earn better money. Due to their educational background, chiropractors can fill that void perfectly. However, they would need to realign (pun intended) their ideological perspective on pharmaceuticals and accept the fact that pharmaceuticals have a place in our society. They won't go away. If chiropractors were trained and certified in the ability to prescribe and manage their patients' pharmaceuticals, it would open up an entirely new practice opportunity for chiropractors and provide the much-needed services of a general practitioner.

This could become the wave of the future for the profession. Of course, chiropractors could continue to call themselves spinal specialists, but I would like to see the profession broaden their scope of practice into a much more widespread base of clinical expertise. However, unless the profession finds agreement within to validate scientifically what they do, it will be a continual uphill struggle.

How To Select A Chiropractic Practitioner

If you are planning to see a chiropractor, ask him (or her) questions like these:

- What causes spinal misalignment and subluxation?
- Could this be another kind of imbalance?
- Is this issue spine-related or organic-related?
- How often will you need to see me for office visits?

It is possible to discover causation, even for spinal and joint pain. Once the cause is discovered, chiropractors can usually put everything back into balance from a structural point of view. But, as in Barbara's case cited above, it is essential to discover the true underlying cause(s). The trick is in the discovery process. As chiropractors, we need to get to know our patients better by asking more questions. As patients, we need to be more responsible for our health by asking more questions.

In a perfect world, the patient should have the opportunity to interview the doctor. Doctors have a great deal of knowledge, but they don't always take the time to help you understand what is out of balance in your body. When you are rushed through the office visit, whether it is a medical office or chiropractic clinic, without having real face-to-face time with your doctor, you miss an important component of medical care: the sense of actually being *cared for*. This is a legitimate and necessary part of healing. If you are uncomfortable with any part of your relation with any of your doctors, find a new one.

WILL MY INSURANCE COVER CHIROPRACTIC CARE?

The answer to this question is almost always yes. Chiropractic care is acknowledged and paid for by every major health care carrier that I know of, including Medicare, which sets the standard for health care delivery, unfortunately.

Sadly, those same carriers do not pay for preventive and/or wellness programs. There has been some movement towards wellness and prevention through flex spending accounts, but these are becoming less and less available to patients. Even the Affordable Care Act does little to support any kind of preventive medicine.

Unfortunately, prevention and wellness is not being taken seriously by insurance companies or the government. Our cultural model of health care is completely oriented toward sickness, symptoms, and diseases instead of health and wellness.

BACK TO BASICS

As a physician, I approach each and every patient as an individual and work to try and understand and treat their specific needs. It sounds simple, but we are complex creatures, with influences from within and from without. My intention is to help them discover why they're not feeling well, following an approach where I acknowledge the interrelations of every system of the body, mind, heart, and spirit. This approach allows me to assist patients in very deep and meaningful ways. I chose chiropractic because I knew it would provide me the most useful port of entry into the health delivery field, one where I could work with patients from a very integrative and holographic approach. It is my intention to begin teaching other physicians what I have learned during my 32 years of doctoring.

(This content should be used for informational purposes only. It does not create a doctor-patient relationship with any reader and should not be construed as medical advice. If you need medical advice, please contact a doctor in your community who can assess the specifics of your situation.)

10

Improving Your Quality of Life With Chiropractic Care

by Shan Twit, D.C.

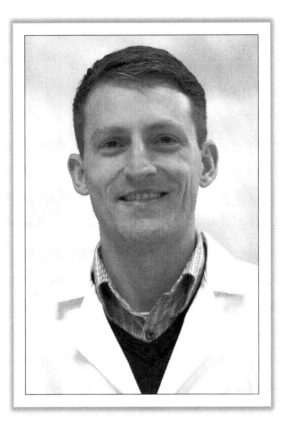

Shan Twit, D.C.
Stamford Chiropractic & Rehab Center
Stamford, Connecticut
www.stamfordchiro.com

Dr. Shan Twit was blessed to having been raised in a chiropractic family and after experiencing what chiropractic care could provide firsthand, he decided to go into the same profession as his father.

After earning a Bachelor's degree in Biology from the University of Wisconsin, Stevens Point, Dr. Twit attended the prestigious Palmer College of Chiropractic in Davenport, IA where he earned his doctorate in Chiropractic. Dr. Twit has been in practice since 2004 and is married to his wife, Nicole.

IMPROVING YOUR QUALITY OF LIFE WITH CHIROPRACTIC CARE

PAIN AND ITS FUNCTION IN YOUR BODY

When most people come to see me, it's usually because they are in pain. Happily, that fact is changing, as people are becoming more proactive when it comes to their health. Patients present to my office with headaches, back pain, neck pain, shoulder pain, poor digestion, migraines, foot pain, and the list goes and on. Chiropractors see people of all ages and with many conditions, but chiropractors are not just back doctors. We're musculoskeletal specialists. We focus on adjusting the entire body in order to help the person improve immune system function, and the best part is that we don't use medication to accomplish that goal.

Pain and discomfort are usually what motivates a person to see a doctor, whether it's a general medical practitioner, a chiropractor, or a dentist. Most people assume if they have pain, there's a problem, which is often the case because pain is the body's way of telling you that something isn't working properly. However, many people also assume that if they don't have symptoms, everything's fine.

It's not that simple.

You could have a serious condition like scoliosis, or even cancer, without experiencing pain. You could have a 90 percent blockage in your blood vessels leading to the heart and be a cardiovascular ticking time bomb waiting to happen and still be pain-free. Every year, many conditions kill millions of people who don't experience any symptoms until it's too late. Some patients find out afterward that the cancer is too advanced or that the carotid artery is 95 percent blocked and they're a stroke waiting to happen!

Pain is just one function of the central nervous system. Pick any nerve in your body. Ninety percent of that nerve's function revolves around communication. The lion's share of that nerve's reason for existence is to transmit electrical impulses from the brain to the shoulder, the kidney, the left foot, or wherever, and then finally complete the circuit back to the brain. This electrical nerve impulse is like water spurting from a hose. If someone steps on the hose, the water stops.

Only 10 percent of that nerve's job is pain sensitivity. Waiting until you have pain is a very reactive way of dealing with your health. Extensive damage could be happening to your body while you're still waiting for a pain signal that won't come. We need to be more proactive about the welfare of our bodies.

The body is amazing and we're still learning more about how it functions every day. The scientific community often acts sure of itself and imagines that it has all the answers. This over-confidence would disappear if people would just look at medical school texts and the way that they change from publication to publication and from year to year. What we "knew" fifty years ago and proclaimed in those textbooks is very different from what we "know" today. To say that we've figured out the body is ludicrous and quite arrogant. For example, many people don't know that just one cubic inch of the brain contains over 10,000 miles of connective tissue. The human brain controls literally billions of chemical impulses every second. If you attached every capillary, artery, and vein end to end in a straight line, that line of blood vessels would reach 60,000 miles. Basically, the human body is so complex and to say we completely understand its every function just isn't true.

No matter what we learn or how much we think we know about the body, the one thing we know for sure is that the central nervous system controls everything. The health of the central nervous system relies heavily on proper curvature within the spine. Without the proper spinal curvature, your body is unable to effectively deal with the force of gravity or to properly absorb the forces applied to it when you lift something or when you slip or fall. The spinal curves act like the shocks and struts of a vehicle: they absorb the forces applied to the weight of your body. When your spine is not functioning the way that it's meant to do, you'll run into problems—and pain.

Everything from the neck down is affected by misalignments of the upper portion of the neck. For example, the *Superman* actor (Christopher Reeve) damaged his spinal column between vertebrae C1 and C2, at the very top portion of his neck. As a result, he became a quadriplegic and lost almost every bodily function. He could only blink his eyes, and he could barely talk. He needed the assistance of an iron lung in order to breathe properly. This is my point: wherever the spine is damaged, everything below that point is affected. But you don't have to have permanent spinal cord damage in order to prevent the brain from properly communicating with the rest of your body. This is especially true when it comes to the upper portion of your neck.

The amount of pressure on a nerve equal to the weight of a dime is enough to reduce the nerve impulse from the brain by up to 60 percent as determined by a study at the University of Colorado.

Waiting until you experience pain or discomfort before seeking the help of a doctor doesn't make much sense either. Up to 40 percent of your immune system can shut down before you're aware there's even an issue in the form of a symptom. That's why being proactive, whether or not you are suffering from symptoms, is the best approach. It's for that same reason we brush our teeth every day despite not having pain. Brushing your teeth is a form of preventative maintenance. If you focus on being proactive about your health, health issues are a lot easier to resolve. Receiving regular chiropractic adjustments, even when you don't have symptoms, is like getting regular oil changes for your car. Almost everything in life requires constant upkeep or maintenance in order to ensure proper function. Your spine is no different.

Pain is a very good motivator—it tells you what to avoid, and which things you should not do. "Whoa, my back hurts. I shouldn't try to lift the box that weighs 40 pounds." "It hurts when I turn my head to the right." However, even though this is an effective and temporary Band-Aid, avoidance of an activity is not the ultimate solution. People are really good at either avoiding the activity or taking a drug to mask the painful symptom. The problem isn't fixed by taking this route and the actual healing is delayed. A better solution is to get rid of the cause of the issue and that's where chiropractic care really shines!

EDUCATION – A PROACTIVE PANACEA

Our educational role is a part of what distinguishes chiropractors from other healers. In Latin, the term "doctor" means "teacher." Therefore, education is one of our first responsibilities. It is the doctor's responsibility to educate the patient about health. One of the most common complaints that bewildered patients express to me is that, "The doctor didn't take the time to explain it to me." Chiropractors pride themselves on the ability to explain the "why" to their patients.

Chiropractors consider the education of our patients to be a critical part of the healing process. This is especially true when we point out that the overall goal of chiropractic care is to boost the immune system, rather than to chase symptoms, which is counterproductive. We teach patients about nutrition and injury prevention, central nervous system health, and the general way that your immune system works. Not only do we help the patient understand how the body works, but we also take the time to demonstrate how the body can work to heal itself. Chiropractic practice is a truly non-invasive, non-pharmaceutical, non-surgical, conservative approach to health.

Chiropractic is based on the fact that the central nervous system controls everything, and we help our patients to strengthen their immune systems from within. Truly, this approach to health care is the most powerful means for improving a person's overall well-being. True wellness does not mean tinkering with the chemicals that your body already produces naturally by adding a synthetic drug to the mix. Healing involves much more than treating the symptoms or turning down the volume on the SOS signals sent by your body, so that your brain doesn't know that your body needs help anymore.

Nor do our patients have to guard themselves against those sinister side effects announced in every miracle drug commercial on television. I find it ironic that the drugs for depression (psychotropics) developed by pharmaceutical companies are associated with a higher risk of suicide for patients. Also, it's amazing that FDA-approved Humira® can give people cancer, yet it's used to treat the symptoms of immune system conditions such as rheumatoid arthritis, colitis, and psoriasis. Chiropractic care works to strengthen your immune system naturally without adding anything foreign to the system. There are many benefits to chiropractic care, but strengthening the immune system is the biggest benefit.

UNDER-CELEBRATED CHIROPRACTIC BENEFITS

Chiropractic care also helps to improve both the patient's strength and range of motion. Our young patients who participate in sports, for example, enjoy a quicker healing time than their teammates who don't receive chiropractic care. The same is true for people injured on the job. In multiple studies done with Workers' Compensation claims across the country, those patients who were treated with chiropractic care returned to work faster than those who used conventional medicine only.

In a study by the *Journal of American Medical Association* (JAMA), it was recommended that patients seek back pain treatment from a chiropractor before pursuing invasive mea-sures like surgery.

There was another study from the medical journal *Spine* that revealed something quite interesting. They stated that "...sufferers of lower back pain all received standard medical care (SMC) and half of the participants additionally received chiropractic care. The researchers found that in SMC plus chiropractic care patients, *73 percent* reported that their pain was completely gone or much better after treatment compared to *just 17 percent* of the SMC group."

Personally, I can attest to the fact that chiropractic care helped me in my own athletic pursuits. I competed in Taekwondo for over 20 years, which led to a great deal of trauma to my head, neck, and upper back. However, I was able to stay competitive in the martial arts because of receiving regular chiropractic adjustments.

In my office, we see parents who bring in their kids to get adjusted. Often they'll say things like "Gosh, Johnny's doing so much better in baseball now that he's getting adjusted. He doesn't get injured as often on the field." Or they'll say, "My daughter doesn't get migraines anymore!"

You might discount some of these stories as anecdotal when you have 5, 10, or even 50 patients sharing these kinds of observations. However, when you see hundreds of patients who tell you the same thing, you know it's true. Chiropractic care results in stronger bodies, improved range of motion, strength, and hand-eye coordination. All of these advantages help the body to stay out of trouble and injuries are far less frequent. Children often show improvement in their overall immune systems and less reliance on medication as a result of getting adjusted. These are just some of the additional benefits of chiropractic care

CAN INFANTS AND SMALL CHILDREN BENEFIT FROM CHIROPRACTIC CARE?

I get this question from my patients quite often, and the answer is a resounding YES! People ask about the safety of chiropractic care for children and even infants and I assure them that chiropractic is very safe for all ages. So far my youngest patient was 37 hours old and my oldest patient was 99 years and 9 months old.

One good way to demonstrate its safety is to review medical malpractice insurance data. Every doctor must carry "med-mal," and the average chiropractor pays approximately $1,500–2,000 or less for medical malpractice insurance. After researching the average medical malpractice insurance premiums for pediatricians, you'll find they might pay anywhere from $10,000 a year on the low end to as high as $50,000 or more depending on where in the country the doctor practices, which I found very interesting.

I can personally attest to the effectiveness of chiropractic care. My father has practiced as a chiropractor in Wisconsin since 1976 and still practices today. I'm one of five kids, and we've all undergone chiropractic care within the first few days of birth and we continue to get regular care. Chiropractic has kept me healthy and my immune system very strong.

My siblings and I were never really sick during our childhood. I myself only missed two days of school from the time that I began elementary school all the way through graduate school—combined. My other siblings have very similar stories. Like most children, we were in contact with kids who were constantly sick with this virus or that bacterial bug. We all went to public schools and were never vaccinated either. That's a testament to what chiropractic care can do.

Literally, I've taken care of hundreds of children under the age of five years. The adjustment procedure for a child is similar to that of an adult adjustment, though it's done with far less force. The adjustment for an infant is a very, very gentle procedure. I wouldn't adjust a college football player in the same way that I would a six-month-old baby, but they both have a spine so they both can get adjusted. Babies deserve the gift of health through chiropractic care just like their parents.

I love when the parents come in saying things like, "I've really noticed how my kids have become so much healthier since coming in to see you," or, "John isn't taking medications anymore."

I recommend chiropractic care for people of all ages because of its safety and efficacy. With children, one of the most striking results is the speed with which they respond and heal. Since they don't typically have the same traumatic history as adults—such as stress, medication use, car accidents, and sports injuries—they tend to heal very quickly.

At what point should chiropractic care begin? Ideally, we like to see infants within hours of their birth but certainly within the first couple months. This will help to jump-start their lives with the right foot forward. They get the advantage of being properly aligned from the get-go. You might be asking yourself, "Why would they be improperly aligned in the first place?" Birth is a very harrowing process.

The birth process is an amazing process to see, but it's also very traumatic to the spine. The baby's spine is twisted and confined within the womb for months and this also places a lot of pressure on the spinal column. The physician must grab the baby's head and will twist and pull the baby through the vaginal canal which exerts a tremendous amount of pressure on the delicate, still growing spine. We know the shape of the birth canal. Considering the size of everything that must come out of that tiny little hole—from the head and neck to the shoulders and hips—even a normal birth is astonishing. There is much resistance and a lot of torque inflicted upon an infant's delicate neck and upper cervical spine. The cervical spine is a very important part of the body. After all of that, the spine can easily become misaligned.

Doing an assessment on the infant certainly doesn't mean that baby will require the same amount of care as mom or dad, though an exam is still a good idea. Just as you will eventually take your little one to the dentist, early chiropractic care can teach your children to be proactive about their health in the future.

Is Chiropractic Care A Forever Thing?

People commonly express the idea that once you've been to a chiropractor, you'll have to keep going for the rest of your life. We teach, preach, and believe that ongoing care is an excellent way to prevent problems in the future. However, patients are not required to do any such thing. The chiropractic police won't be calling on you to issue a ticket for alignment infractions. Nevertheless, ongoing chiropractic care is a practical step in the right direction.

A classic example of this approach can be found inside the glove compartment of your car. If you check the owner's manual of your new vehicle, you'll find a book that describes the type of maintenance schedule to follow. Carmakers are so serious about this that if you fail to follow their very specific guidelines, they won't warranty your vehicle. Old oil can tear up an engine. Misaligned wheels tear up tires and turn your vehicle into a danger on the streets. Maintenance preserves the vehicle, lowers the overall costs, and increases the safety margin for you and your passengers. Life requires maintenance.

Even if a small amount of rust on the car door doesn't immediately affect the door, it may spread and, 10 years later, when you try to open the door, it falls off. You should take your car in for tire rotations and alignment, which affects the function of the vehicle. You should schedule oil changes. You should brush your teeth, and certainly you should bathe. All of these things should be done proactively and most of us instinctively understand the benefits of engaging in all of these responsible tasks. Sadly, when it comes to our bodies, many people still tend to follow the paradigm dictated by western medical minds. We show up at the clinic when we are sick or are in pain. In the chiropractic field, we want to prevent illness, rather than treating it after the fact.

Your central nervous system, which is the brain and the spinal cord, doesn't control just a few things. It controls everything. Your heart and your lungs are important, but they are controlled by your central nervous system - just like every other system in your entire body. The brain and spinal cord are responsible for the functioning of more than 75 trillion cells in your body. These include your teeth, hair, skin, skeletal muscles, reproductive organs, and even your digestion. Even though we live in an amazing technological era that provides available replacement parts for nearly every one of your organs that fails to function, you only get one brain and one spinal cord. Think about that. *You cannot replace your central nervous system. And the only two structures in the body which are housed and protected by solid bone are the brain and the spinal cord.* That describes the critical nature of the central nervous system, and the importance of preventative maintenance care for your long-term health and well-being.

I'm happy to report that more than 90 percent of my patients choose lifetime care because they understand the benefit of prevention. Long after the pain has passed, they choose to continue chiropractic care under a preventive, wellness-based approach. After the symptoms have vanished, they don't ever want to repeat the pain that brought them through the door in the first place. When our patients return for regular care, this means that we have successfully relayed the most important message that we have to share with our patients.

HOW OFTEN MUST PATIENTS RETURN FOR MAINTENANCE CARE?

Once the patient returns to pre-injury status—normal range of motion, strength, and overall immune system health—the vast majority of my patients understand that prevention is worth that continuing effort. That maintenance routine probably means a once-a-month visit, which is average for most adults. In some cases it's more frequent, depending upon the situation, because a specific chronic issue may require an adjustment once every two to three weeks for an extended period of time. For young children, it's usually much less frequent because they snap back into shape much more quickly and don't have the same history as the adult patient.

This is just a general idea of what to expect and everyone's circumstances are different.

A five-month-old can't really tell his case history to a chiropractor in the same way as an adult can. So you rely quite heavily on what the parents say and their reactions to the care. In summary, the lifestyle or maintenance care frequency for children is far less than the schedule laid out for an adult, because kids respond so quickly.

It is my hope, and the hope of most chiropractic providers, to change the paradigm as it relates to the way our society looks at health. My perspective is unique, I think, because of my father. After nearly 40 years of practice, he has seen all sorts of changes in social perception about the chiropractic profession. He's observed that perception change from chiropractors being viewed as quacks who weren't "real" doctors to chiropractors being accepted as respected members of the medical community. Many second- and third-generation chiropractors will agree with me on that, having been exposed to the chiropractic lifestyle their entire lives.

People used to have some apprehension about chiropractic work because they didn't understand it. It's also not a surprise when those sentiments come from the individual who's never been to a chiropractor. That's like saying you can't have spicy food despite never having tried it. Additionally, there was an ongoing feud between the medical paradigm and the homeopathic paradigm, into which chiropractic fits. Nor did it help that for many years chiropractic care wasn't covered by insurance policies. Today however the vast majority of private insurance companies now provide some type of chiropractic care coverage. Medicare and Medicaid cover chiropractic care as well which only adds to the credibility of the profession. Veterans also have access to chiropractic care in VA hospitals across the country.

Personally, I adhere to a different philosophy when it comes to insurance coverage. I believe that, at the end of the day, the individual is solely responsible for his or her health. I also believe that doctors should make care affordable so that the masses can enjoy the benefits of chiropractic. To that extent, I'm not personally in-network with any insurance company, and all of my patients pay out-of-pocket for a specific reason: I choose not to answer to an insurance company. Instead, I like to answer directly to the patient. Instead of offering care based on what an insurance company will cover, I give my patients what they need and deserve and I keep it affordable. It's for this reason I have many unemployed patients and also people that come to visit me from out-of-state. However, it's still valuable and reassuring to some people that their insurance policy will cover chiropractic care if they choose to use it.

Patient perceptions are changing in many ways. At the time of this publication, I will have been in practice for 10 1/2 years. I've noticed people coming in more often simply because they want to get evaluated by a chiropractor and not only because they were in a recent car accident or because of a painful symptom. The initial conversation goes something like this: "You know my friend comes to see you for her low back pain. I really don't have any symptoms, but I just want to get checked by a chiropractor."

It's refreshing to see people concerned about the health of their overall immune system. They want to know if they are doing well from a biomechanical and structural point of view.

Being proactive is definitely the way to go and I sense the paradigm shifting in this regard.

YOUR FIRST VISIT

If you've never been to a chiropractor, you may think the sound of the word "adjustment" seems ominous. It's not as scary when you already know what usually happens during your first visit. It's for this reason that I recommend that patients bring in their spouses so they can see their loved ones receive an adjustment firsthand.

Long before we get to the actual adjustment, I sit down with each patient to get to know the person through a consultation. When Joe Smith walks into my office, I don't know anything about him. I don't know what he's feeling, nor am I sure if he is able to effectively relate his symptoms to me. Until I begin the consultation, I don't know his history in terms of injuries or the medications that he currently takes or anything else that Joe does in his life.

After the consultation I perform an exam. The exam includes orthopedic tests, taking the patient's vitals, observational posture analysis, neurological tests and range of motion testing. When examining the patient's posture I check to see if his weight is evenly distributed between the left and right side of the body. It's like the alignment of a car—I want to see if all of the important things are balanced. I want to look at the gait cycle and the way the patient walks, to see if he favors one side over the other. Remember, proper structure and alignment equals proper function.

After the consultation and exam it's necessary to analyze an x-ray and take the measurements to determine which vertebrae are misaligned. The term chiropractors use to describe the misaligned vertebrae is the *subluxation complex*. A *subluxation* is when a joint in the body is fixated or "stuck" out of alignment. This misalignment compromises the brain's ability to communicate with the rest of the body. If there is nerve pressure anywhere along the length of the spine, this is like the stepping on the hose analogy: it cuts off the flow. In the human body, this equates to reducing nerve flow which compromises the immune system. The adjustment removes the nerve interference and this alleviates the pain but more importantly improves your function.

THE GONSTEAD METHOD OF ADJUSTMENT

The Gonstead method was invented by Dr. Clarence Gonstead. He was a mechanical engineer and pilot, who developed one of the most successful practices in the United States in the middle part of the 20th century. He and his wife initially practiced above a bank in the small town of Mount Horeb, Wisconsin.

Doctor Gonstead was producing results with his patients that no other doctors could produce; the word of his successful treatments spread like wildfire. People would line up in his reception room, out into the hallway, out onto the sidewalk, and down the street. Gonstead would adjust up to 250 patients per day and it wasn't unusual for him to work 18–20 hours per day, 6 ½ days per week. Ultimately, he built a 29,000 square foot clinic. Then, he built a hotel next to the clinic to accommodate for the overflow of patients. Later, he constructed an airstrip on the one side of the building, so that out-of-state and out-of-country patients could fly in to Mount Horeb, Wisconsin which, at the time, was a small town of about 1,500 people.

Prior to the internet age, his successes were broadcast by word of mouth. His work was based upon the analysis of an X-ray and how the misaligned vertebrae within the spine irritated the discs, which could cause neurological problems. He would look at the patient's X-ray and compare it to that of a normal healthy spine. Then, he would explain his findings to the patient in what is called the Report of Findings (ROF).

Dr. Gonstead was able to analyze an X-ray and determine the location of these misalignments within the spine. His technique was very objective—it wasn't based upon hunches or guesses, or even the patients' feelings or doctors' thoughts. It was based entirely on the information displayed by the exam and the X-ray. Period. His technique is just as consistently reliable today as it was when Dr. Gonstead was actively in practice.

I use the same technique to determine the necessary level of treatment. For the adjustment itself, I use my hands. Chiropractic means "practice with your hands." Other doctors use a tool called an Activator to accomplish a high-speed, low-force adjustment. Some chiropractors will use the tool for any number of reasons, perhaps because they don't know if they have the necessary hand strength and/or skill to do the adjustment by hand, or because their geriatric patients require soft handling. I use my hands, as do the vast majority of the chiropractors in the country. Over the years and with practice, a good chiropractor's hands develop the tactile sensitivity and the palpation skills that a tool can never duplicate.

Depending on the situation, in addition to a plain film radiograph (x-ray), there may be a need for an MRI to rule out a possible disc herniation. It's possible to find a chiropractor who won't require X-rays, but those doctors are not among the majority.

I attended the Palmer College of Chiropractic, located in Davenport, Iowa. It was the first chiropractic college, begun in 1895, and is still the largest and longest-standing university for chiropractic in the United States. The standard protocol taught at Palmer is that chiropractors first engage the patient in a consultation and then do an exam. Then the doctor would proceed based upon those exam findings. An X-ray is necessary if the patient has radiculopathy (numbness) or paresthesia (tingling going down the extremities). X-rays are also necessary if the patient has lost muscle strength, shows a severely diminished range of motion, and/or is in pain. I take an X-ray of almost every patient unless the patient is an infant or if he brings in his own X-rays.

The reason for requiring an X-ray is simple and is very similar to the analogy of fixing a vehicle. If you want to fix the engine of a car, you don't simply wash and wax it; you pop the hood. When you pop the hood, you can see the engine. By doing so you'll know if it's a battery that needs replacing instead of maybe a bad starter. Proceeding without looking is just guesswork. I'm not going to guess with my patients.

When I look at the X-ray, first I will want to see the curvature of the spine and the overall alignment. Secondly, I need to rule out pathology. I need to verify that this person is not suffering from any conditions that would be better addressed by an MD: gall stones, kidney stones, cancer, cysts, or aneurysms are seen often enough to warrant taking a film. If a patient insists that he/she doesn't want an x-ray no matter what, then I may have to refer him or her to another health care provider.

Finally, I want to rule out fractures. Let's say that Mrs. Jones comes in and says, "I have some pain in my mid-back. It hurts when I breathe in. It's sharp." If she has a fracture of the fifth rib on the right and I proceed to adjust T5, which is the fifth thoracic vertebrae which attaches to the fifth rib head, I could be making the problem much worse. I've always taken the position that chiropractic care is either specific or it's nothing. We take an X-ray to be more specific and to be more effective with the adjustment, it's really that simple.

I also recommend that patients get a weight-bearing, or standing, X-ray. The same is true with MRIs. Imagine that Mrs. Jones' doctor has ordered an MRI. Dr. Smith thinks that Mrs. Jones has a disc herniation at L5. He sends her out for an MRI and the technicians create the images while she's supine, or lying on her back.

In this situation, the problem is that Mrs. Jones' disc herniation might not appear prominently while she's lying down. However, when she's standing, her spine is vertical. As gravity puts more pressure on that disc, it makes the problem more evident. A disc herniation that is mild when the person is lying down could be much more severe and obvious when she is standing. I must see the bigger picture of the activity in the patient's spine if I'm supposed to do what's best for the patient.

THE CHIROPRACTIC ADVANTAGE

Many patients don't realize that chiropractors are real doctors. The DC behind our names stands for "Doctor of Chiropractic," just as DO stands for "Doctor of Osteopathy," and MD stands for "Medical Doctor." There are two basic philosophies or paradigms in patient treatment: homeopathic and allopathic. Homeopathic includes acupuncture, chiropractic, and massage. Allopathic includes pharmaceutical drugs and surgery.

In my opinion, taking a more homeopathic approach to health is the best method. Chiropractic doesn't put anything into the system or take anything out. Instead, by removing nerve interference, we allow your marvelous body to heal itself. As they say, the body doesn't need any help, it just needs a lack of interference. That's the biggest difference between the homeopathic and allopathic approach.

Also, chiropractors go to school for about three years and four months before they take board exams to become licensed. For the first two to two-and-a-half years of schooling, there's very little difference between medical and chiropractic classes which include: neuroanatomy, diagnosis, spinal anatomy, pathology, physiology, radiology, and microbiology—just to name a few. Once licensed, the chiropractor must obtain the required continuing education credits in order to maintain their licensure as well as carry adequate medical malpractice insurance. After high school I went to undergraduate college for four years to earn my Bachelor's degree in biology. Then I attended another four years at Palmer College of Chiropractic before earning my doctorate in chiropractic.

At the time this book goes to press I'm currently practicing in Connecticut, which requires chiropractors to pass four board exams, along with a fifth: physiotherapy—in order get licensed to practice. Every two years, I have to take 48 hours of continuing education to keep my license.

Ultimately, it's the philosophy of the doctor that dictates the treatment options for the patient. If your doctor believes that health comes from the outside in, he will likely give you drugs to solve your problem, or provide symptom relief by removing the "problem" like getting a cholecystectomy (surgical removal of the gallbladder.) If your doctor's philosophy says that health comes from the inside out, he will take different steps. "I'm going to talk to you about nutrition," he will say. "I'm going to talk to you about posture, your amazing central nervous system, and the way it functions. I'm also going to make some dietary recommendations for you. Health and healing comes from within."

It is not just a matter of opinion that chiropractic care can make a profound difference in peoples' lives. There was a large seven-year study[1] posted by The Journal of Physiological and Manipulative Therapeutics (JMPT), involving over 70,000 people over a seven-year period. Researchers found that patients whose primary health care provider was a chiropractor, rather than an MD, used 85 percent less medications and had 62 percent fewer hospital admissions. That's pretty powerful.

Another case study[2], done by a medical doctor in Chicago (Bakris), was posted on WebMD. This study focused on the efficiency and effectiveness of chiropractic adjustments on high blood pressure. The subjects were divided into two groups: one group was given a fake adjustment, and the other group actually received a real chiropractic adjustment of the upper cervical vertebrae (called the Atlas), which is the first cervical vertebrae in your neck at the base of your skull. The group that received the real adjustment showed up to a 14-point systolic drop in blood pressure, which were better results than those patients who took the blood pressure-lowering medications. The atlas adjustment is so effective because 50 percent of your neck's rotation occurs around the atlas. If it's misaligned, it can affect blood pressure by compressing onto the vagus nerve, which is one of the most important nerves in the entire human body.

The vagus nerve, your tenth cranial nerve, feeds directly into your heart and many of the organs below the heart. The study found that those people with an upper cervical misalignment (compressing the vasculature and the nerve supply of the upper portion of the neck) had higher blood pressure. When the atlas was realigned properly to reduce pressure on the vagus nerve, the blood pressure dropped by up to 14 points. This was a very powerful study! So despite the lack of big pharma advertising dollars to back up our message, despite the lack of chiropractic commercials or lobbying money, chiropractors have the most effective advertising tool on the planet: *patient referrals* and *results*.

The chiropractic approach sets our discipline apart from other health care providers. I firmly believe that our work is one of the most effective ways to offer help to our patients. We have the advantage of being tuned in to the body in a different way—a *proactive* way—and it translates into better health and happiness for our patients.

(This content should be used for informational purposes only. It does not create a doctor-patient relationship with any reader and should not be construed as medical advice. If you need medical advice, please contact a doctor in your community who can assess the specifics of your situation.)

References:

[1]"Clinical Utilization and Cost Outcomes From an Integrative Medicine Independent Physician Association: An Additional 3-Year Update" *Journal of Manipulative and Physiological Therapeutics (JMPT)*: Volume 30, Issue 4, May, 2007, Pages 263-269. http://www.jmptonline.org/article/S0161-4754(07)00076-0/abstract

[2]"Chiropractic Cuts Blood Pressure: Study Finds Special 'Atlas Adjustment' Lowers Blood Pressure" *WebMD Health.*: March,16 2007 http://www.webmd.com/hypertension-high-blood-pressure/news/20070316/chiropractic-cuts-blood-pressure.

Made in the USA
Lexington, KY
29 January 2015